CONTINUING CARE

A multidisciplinary approach to discharge planning

Edited by

KATHLEEN M. McKEEHAN, R.N., M.S.

Formerly Continuing Care Coordinator, Boston Hospital for Women, Division of the Affiliated Hospital Center, Inc. (now known as Brigham and Women's Hospital), Boston, Massachusetts

Instructional design by

Barbara R. Pollack

With **46** *illustrations*

The C. V. Mosby Company

ST. LOUIS • TORONTO • LONDON 1981

Printed in the United States of America

The C. V. Mosby Company
11830 Westline Industrial Drive, St. Louis, Missouri 63141

Library of Congress Cataloging in Publication Data

Main entry under title:

Continuing care.

Bibliography: p.
Includes index.
1. Hospitals—Admission and discharge.
2. Hospitals—After care—Planning. 3. Health care teams. I. McKeehan, Kathleen M., 1940- [DNLM: 1. After care. 2. Patient discharge. 3. Patient care planning. WX158 C762]
RA971.8.C68 362.1′1′0685 80-22653
ISBN 0-8016-3285-4

C/M/M 9 8 7 6 5 4 3 2 1 05/B/598

Contributors

Sandra Austin, R.N., B.S.

Continuing Care Coordinator,
Boston City Hospital,
Boston Massachusetts

Louise W. Brine, R.N.

Formerly Administrator of the Elm Hill Nursing Home, Boston, Massachusetts; Graduate of Notre Dame Academy, Roxbury, Massachusetts, and Boston City Hospital School of Nursing, Boston, Massachusetts

Kathleen Thompson Burke, R.N., M.S.

Instructor of Nursing,
Salem State College,
Salem, Massachusetts;
formerly Coordinated Home Care Coordinator, Boston Visiting Nurse Association, Boston, Massachusetts

Robert D. Emerman, M.B.A.

Vice-President for Administrative Services, Affiliated Hospital Center, Inc. (now known as Brigham and Women's Hospital), Boston, Massachusetts

Lucy Feild, R.N., M.S.

Assistant Professor of Nursing,
Boston University;
formerly Assistant Head Nurse,
Renal Transplant Unit,
Peter Bent Brigham Hospital,
Division of the Affiliated Hospital Center, Inc. (now known as Brigham and Women's Hospital), Boston, Massachusetts

Jennifer R. Frost

Graphics Assistant,
Educational Resources Department,
Boston Hospital for Women,
Division of the Affiliated Hospital Center, Inc. (now known as Brigham and Women's Hospital), Boston, Massachusetts

Patricia Gleason-Claydon, R.D., M.S.

Associate Director,
Department of Dietetics and Nutrition,
Boston Hospital for Women,
Division of the Affiliated Hospital Center, Inc. (now known as Brigham and Women's Hospital), Boston, Massachusetts

Lillian Weiner Gray, M.S., C.C.C.

Director of Speech-Language Pathology,
Massachusetts Rehabilitation Hospital,
Boston, Massachusetts

Patricia M. Kearney, R.D., M.Ed.

Nutritionist for Ambulatory and Community Health Services,
Boston Hospital for Women,
Division of the Affiliated Hospital Center, Inc. (now known as Brigham and Women's Hospital), Boston, Massachusetts

Margaret E. LaMontagne, R.N., M.S., J.D.

Associate Director of Nursing and Associate Director for Parkway Administration, Boston Hospital for Women, Division of the Affiliated Hospital Center, Inc. (now known as Brigham and Women's Hospital), Boston, Massachusetts

Robert J. Master, M.D.

Medical Director, Uphams Corner Health Center; Assistant Professor, Department of Socio-Medical Sciences and Community Medicine, Boston University School of Medicine, Boston, Massachusetts

Kathleen M. McKeehan, R.N., M.S.

Student, Ph.D. Program in Nursing, Frances Payne Bolton School of Nursing, Case Western Reserve University, Cleveland, Ohio;
formerly Continuing Care Coordinator, Boston Hospital for Women, Division of the Affiliated Hospital Center, Inc. (now known as Brigham and Women's Hospital); formerly Staff Nurse, Transfer Office, Massachusetts General Hospital, Boston, Massachusetts

Elizabeth J. Nevel, R.N., M.S.

Assistant Continuing Care Coordinator, Boston Hospital for Women, Division of the Affiliated Hospital Center, Inc. (now known as Brigham and Women's Hospital), Boston, Massachusetts

Janet Papile O'Day, R.N., M.S., M.P.H.

Director of Continuing Care Department, Carney Hospital, Boston, Massachusetts

Jean Oulund Peteet, R.P.T., B.S.

Director of Physical Therapy, Massachusetts Rehabilitation Hospital, Boston, Massachusetts

Barbara R. Pollack, M.Ed.

Director of Educational Resources Department, Boston Hospital for Women, Division of the Affiliated Hospital Center, Inc. (now known as Brigham and Women's Hospital), Boston, Massachusetts

C. David Rison

Graphics Designer, Educational Resources Department, Boston Hospital for Women, Division of the Affiliated Hospital Center, Inc. (now known as Brigham and Women's Hospital), Boston, Massachusetts

Guitelle H. Sandman, A.C.S.W., M.S.W.

Chief of Oncology Social Work Services, Boston Hospital for Women, Division of the Affiliated Hospital Center, Inc. (now known as Brigham and Women's Hospital), Boston, Massachusetts

Michael J. Steinhauer, O.T.R., B.S.

Medical Graduate Student, Northwestern University Medical School, Chicago, Illinois; formerly Director, Occupational Therapy Services, Senior Home Care Services, Boston, Massachusetts

Cynthia MacDonald Walsh, R.N., B.S.N.

Staff Nurse, Continuing Care Department, Carney Hospital, Boston, Massachusetts

To

CLIENTS/PATIENTS

and to

Providers of health care who have taken the risk to release territorial barriers and work together as colleagues in health care planning teams

Foreword

A patient's perspective of discharge planning

I am Ruth Galloway, age 65. I have been happily married for 40 years, and I am the mother of three children, David, Michael, and Anne. We are proud of them; they of us. I taught junior high school students in New Jersey for 22 years, a grand and compelling experience. We published a monthly magazine, produced plays, and wrote poetry while learning grammar, spelling, and English literature. These were the halcyon days, but like splendor in the grass, they came to an end. As my health problems began, so did my nightmare.

The first signs of my physical breakdown involved a fierce thirst, exhaustion, and a staggering walk. One bitterly cold, snowy day, I decided not to wait for the bus and walked the two miles home. I had always been strong and healthy. When I was almost home, a surge of illness attacked me as I was passing a doctor's office. I walked into the office immediately. A personable young man examined me. He was an obstetrician, a somewhat surprised one! Arriving home, I found my daughter, Anne, home from her day at junior college. "Anne, doll, I'm going to lie down for a half hour. Call me. I've papers to correct and dinner to start." Later, they were unable to arouse me. The coma lasted three days, and I awakened to species of bottles, jars, pans—all the implements necessary for the care of a "patient."

My recovery progressed. I was put on a strict diet, shown how to use a needle for daily insulin shots, and given pamphlets, menus, advice, and best wishes. That was the end; there was no follow-up when I returned home. It was rather like being in limbo. I returned to teaching, and everybody was pleased. After all, happiness is a sometime thing.

Retirement came at 57 years of age. I was plain tired of staying up until three or four in the morning, correcting papers. I wanted a rest. The day after my husband retired at the age of 65, I had a paralytic stroke on my entire right side. More hospitalizations and pain. Progress was rather slow, since there was very little of my physical being that remained active. I was quite helpless. My husband did his best to help me.

At long last, on the advice of my doctor, I was taken to a nursing home, where

I remained for six months. It was highly reputed, but to me it was a place for the helpless who slowly begin to die. I had no freedom, no voice, no ideas that I could express. I lay there in that bed, "your home," fed, bathed, and under constant sedation. I was out in the fresh air only six times in six months. I held up my arms—the only physical therapy I received. It was assumed that I had brain damage and that I was going to die—a lost cause. I cried to go home. There were appalling nightmares and hallucinations I can still remember. There was no planning for the future with anyone. I became very bitter.

Finally, my family was given the news that I probably had only two weeks to live. Refusing to accept this news, my daughter appeared on the scene in a few days with an ambulance. I was driven to her home, where my husband, Burt, and I lived for seven months. To say I was discharged from the nursing home would be ludicrous. It was felt by the staff that I should die there. We left with bottles of pills and nothing else.

After two days in my daughter's home, I lapsed into another coma, which led to another ride and another hospital. This coma lasted five days. The care I received was superb. After ten days I was ready for discharge and in better physical and mental health than I had been in years. A good laugh is a beautiful thing, and I was laughing. This time I was allowed to express my feelings and wishes about my plans on discharge. Everyone helped and advised, letting me take part in everything. We discussed what would happen to me when I returned home and what care I would receive. The nurse coordinating my discharge with me arranged for a home health aide to care for me from 8:00 A.M. to 12 noon five days a week. A visiting nurse appeared about every ten days to check my progress, and a physical therapist came within a week to start my exercises with me. A wheelchair and hospital bed completed the setup for the return to life and living.

This all happened two years ago. At that time it was impossible for me to walk. Once a month I went to the hospital to see my doctor. It was astonishing how everyone sincerely cared. In the summer we bought one of those outside pools. My son-in-law came in with me, and I began to swim. By the fall my doctor told me that I was ready for gait training and made arrangements with the physical therapy department. It seems so long ago, buying my first pair of shoes after so many months. The nurse coordinating my discharge with me suggested where I could go for shoes and a brace. All the various people who cared for me worked together at the hospital, contacting me and my family before any decisions were made. The therapists were real warriors, and almost saints. In this hospital you work hard, and your therapist works harder. She never lets you down; you can't let her down. When she tells you to do exercises at home, you do them as if she were there. The therapists have stamina, great hearts, patience, and self-control, and they are dedicated to their patients. They never say, "You're not going to walk again." My therapist knew it would take time, and it did.

I had two more admissions to the hospital—for a bleeding ulcer on my toe.

The doctor thought the toe would have to be amputated, but great care was taken, and it healed. Since I was coming into the hospital for therapy twice a week, it was always possible for the doctor to check me. I was never neglected and always had instructions on what to do when I was at home.

Altogether I have been admitted to and discharged from the hospital five times. I know the emotions and wish to make a few comments with regard to *true* discharge planning.

At the time of each discharge what I wanted most was the feeling that this was not the end of contact with those who had assisted me in every known way—physically and mentally—to prepare me for discharge. No more planned, controlled environment—what a terrifying thought. One longs to be with one's loved ones at home, but at the same time one chooses not to be a burden. Therein lie the ultimate fear and insecurity—being a burden. No such fear was mine when I left the community hospital. My doctor, nurses, therapists, social worker, and discharge planning nurse-consultant all cooperated and planned *with* me and *for* me. My husband and daughter were made a part of all the plans. Everything was arranged, and the support of the visiting nurse, aide, and physical therapist continued at home for six months. All this discharge planning was done in order to prevent my collapsing into a chair to watch television all day—sinking into a rut. Perhaps if this support had been given when I was in the nursing home, I might be running now, or at least *jogging*. I might never have had the fear, despair, and constant feeling of being nothing but a vegetable.

One who has health problems of any nature should almost immediately realize that professional help is needed, not only for an analysis of the particular problem, but for the direction and guidance that should eventually lead to good results. I sought help from the professionals because they knew what was wrong and how to secure answers. After not moving my body independently for a year, I began to recover. From a chair I began to learn how to use my body, faithfully, tediously, and laboriously, exercising daily—even on Sundays. It was a delight to go to the outpatient therapy sessions. The therapists, with their years of training, are unbelievable. I tried never to disappoint them—nurses, doctor, therapists, social worker. I was more than grateful—I loved them. They are the ones who helped me to walk, swim, feed myself, write, dress, bathe myself, and travel—but I still need them until I can dance and run. I am a human, living being, active, loving, still striving for more. I needed professional help to be normal, if there is such a thing as normal. I asked for the help, and they gave it willingly. *Somebody at the Top* likes me, along with my family and all those beautiful health care professionals.

Ruth Galloway

Preface

Discharge planning is one of the most important elements in the delivery of health care today. It is beginning to encompass a very specialized body of knowledge because of increased emphasis on continuity of patient care and the rigorous monitoring of health care by regulatory agencies and third party payers. It is important to stress that throughout this book discharge planning is viewed as only one of many elements in the overall delivery of care and not as a separate entity. The purpose of this book is to analyze this element and offer guidelines so that health care providers from various disciplines can *integrate* discharge planning into the delivery of their professional services.

The philosophy that provides the foundation for this book is twofold: (1) that every patient has a *right* to quality discharge planning and (2) that primary providers from various health care disciplines are *accountable* to that right and have a *responsibility* to integrate discharge planning into their delivery of care. In view of this philosophy, primary providers should have available to them consultants who are educated and experienced in the area of discharge planning.

The aim of this book is to offer a distinct approach to discharge planning. It provides a specific framework that addresses itself to the *scope* of discharge planning, the *structure* involved in the steps of the discharge planning process, *strategies* in implementing a discharge planning program, *management practices* in discharge planning, and *perspectives* of the roles of primary health care providers from multiple disciplines as they plan discharge with their patients and when appropriate as they serve as consultants in discharge planning programs.

The book is designed to offer specific guidelines to individuals directly involved in creating and implementing discharge planning programs. It also offers students from various disciplines an opportunity to view what will be expected of them as they practice their professional roles in health care delivery teams.

All of us have much to learn in this ever changing society that affects the delivery of our health care. It cannot be emphasized enough that one of the most important sources of our learning is feedback from the patients we serve. This book is dedicated to them, and the foreword was written by a patient because we believe that patients are the purpose of our professional existence. Discharge planning is that phase in a patient's life when separation becomes a prime issue. This separation often includes a parting from both environments and relationships. As professional colleagues, we have a responsibility to patients and one another in making the discharge planning process a supportive, meaningful experience.

The contributors to this book were carefully chosen because of their knowledge, competence, and leadership in the area of discharge planning. They were all located in Massachusetts because that was the first state in the country to have formal regulations governing discharge planning practices in acute hospital settings. The regulations, which were passed in August, 1971, can be found in Appendix C.

The model suggested in Chapter 1 regarding implementation of a discharge planning program has been successfully utilized for over nine years. As editor of this book, I believe it is important to point out that my experience over the past 11 years has involved working in discharge planning programs that have been located both in a social service department and in a nursing department of a large teaching general hospital and a specialty hospital. Regardless of the type of hospital, size of hospital, or department in the hospital where the discharge planning program is located, the principles remain the same. It is not the intention of this book to specify in what department discharge planning programs should be located. The placement of a discharge planning program often depends on the traditions and political environment of the institution. They can have either a positive or a negative impact on a program. It is important that a discharge planning program be located within the department that can offer to the patient and health care providers the greatest opportunity to work harmoniously and effectively together. The reader is encouraged to analyze the information offered in this book, test it, and generate new knowledge that hopefully will be shared.

There are two terms used throughout the book that I would like to take the opportunity to operationally define. First, *discharge planning* is defined as the process of activities that involve the patient and a team of individuals from various disciplines working together to facilitate the transition of that patient from one environment to another. The transitional environments are usually hospitals, nursing homes, or the patient's community home (including the home of a significant other person). Second, the term *patient* is utilized in its broadest sense and encompasses not only the sick individual but the *client* who takes a more active role in participating in his own discharge planning process.

I am indebted to many individuals for helping to make this book possible. In particular I would like to thank Ellen W. Jones, M.P.H., and Paul M. Densen, Sc.D., special leaders in the area of patient assessment and classification in discharge planning; the administration of Boston Hospital for Women for providing a free and creative environment in which to test the conceptual framework offered in this book; the staff and patients at Boston Hospital for Women and Massachusetts General Hospital for allowing me the opportunity to work with and for them; the Boston Regional Continuing Care Nurses' Association for providing an educational environment and a support system that greatly enhanced my development; Marjory Gordon, R.N., Ph.D., for her encouragement to pursue my academic career; faculty at Frances Payne Bolton School of Nursing, Case Western Reserve University; Ruth Anderson, R.N., Ph.D., Virginia Boardman, R.N., Ph.D., and Rosemary Ellis, R.N., Ph.D., for generously sharing their insights and time; Gretchen Crawford, R.N., Ph.D., my jogging partner, for helping me to choose to continue to "run" with my academic life; Joae Graham Brooks, R.N., M.D., for helping me believe that this book could be a reality; and our typists, Betty Ray, Eleanor Watson, and Jeannette Kaufman, for their unending patience and endurance.

I wish to express a special thank-you to my colleagues from both nursing and other disciplines who provided the opportunity for me to work side by side with them as a team member in the delivery of health care. This experience more than any other has had the greatest impact on my professional growth.

Kathleen M. McKeehan

Contents

SECTION THREE

IMPLEMENTATION OF THE DISCHARGE PLANNING PROCESS

SECTION ONE

Organization development

Organization development is described by Bennis as "a response to change, a complex educational strategy intended to change the beliefs, attitudes, values, and structure of organizations so that they can better adapt to new technologies, markets, and challenges, and the dizzying rate of change itself."[1] The accelerated flow of movement due to changes in the delivery of health care has caused many providers to struggle for identity and existence. Discharge planning is one of the fastest-moving areas of health care concentration. As health care providers, we often become creators and victims of our own changes in the delivery of care. To some providers, discharge planning is a new pressure in the changing health scene, and therefore they feel victimized by regulations forcing them to provide a service in a specific way within a defined period of time. To others, formal discharge planning programs are a welcome catalyst for an increase in the quality of health care delivery.

Pierre Teilhard de Chardin once wrote: "If we had to choose between a total process of evolution and a state of complete fixity, that is to say between two absolutes—everything incessantly in motion, or everything forever immovable—we should be bound to choose the first."[2]

Section One is designed to provide a base for the establishment of discharge planning programs and departments. It begins with a conceptual framework that looks at the scope, structure, and implementation of the discharge planning process. Chapter 2 places discharge planning as a priority within hospital administration. Chapter 3 offers specific educational techniques to help the reader educate health care providers from various disciplines to their role in the discharge planning process. The section concludes in Chapter 4 by illustrating how discharge planning consultants can organize to form a supportive network for purposes of personal development and productive political action.

REFERENCES

1. Bennis, W. G.: Organization development: its nature, origins, and prospects, Reading, Mass., Addison-Wesley Publishing Co., p. 2.
2. Teilhard de Chardin, Pierre: The future of man, New York, 1964, Harper & Row, Publishers, p. 12.

CHAPTER 1

Conceptual framework for discharge planning

KATHLEEN M. McKEEHAN

As health care providers, we are responsible to help individuals formulate a personal definition of health. Once the definition has evolved, our role continues as we motivate them to set health as a goal and to develop life patterns that make possible the attainment of this goal. Health is defined to include both the process of fruitful living and meaningful dying. Discharge planning programs exist to provide a vehicle for health care providers from multiple disciplines to work together with the patient to attain the patient's defined goal of health.

The purpose of this chapter is to offer a conceptual framework that organizes components pertaining to the area of discharge planning. The framework consists of three major components: (1) a description of the scope of discharge planning, (2) an explanation of basic steps that comprise the process of discharge planning, and (3) the suggestion of a model through which a discharge planning program can be implemented.

Discharge planning is defined as *the process of activities that involve the patient and a team of individuals from various disciplines working together to facilitate the transition of that patient from one environment to another*. The transitional environments are usually hospitals, nursing homes, or the patient's community home (including the home of a significant other person). The difference between a discharge planning program and a discharge planning department should be explained. A *program* refers to the specific philosophy, goals, and objectives an institution develops in order to carry out the steps of the discharge planning process. A *department* refers to the unit of individuals primarily responsible for facilitating the program. For example, discharge planning consultants would be located within a department.

Rationale for discharge planning has a twofold premise: continuity of care and cost effectiveness. Continuity of care is the term applied to the coordinated deliv-

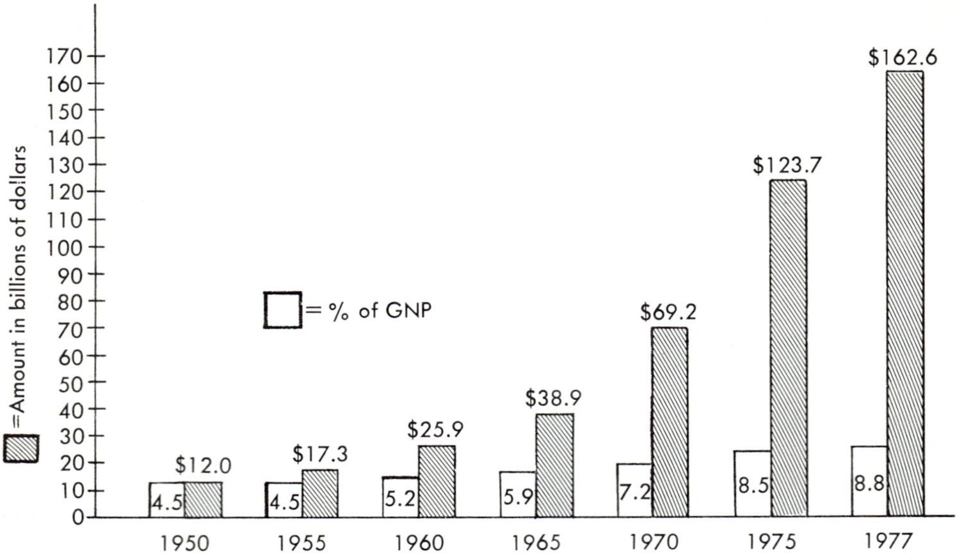

Fig. 1-1. National health expenditures, 1950 to 1977. (From Gibson, R. M., and Fischer, C. R.: National health expenditures, fiscal year 1977, Social Security Bulletin 3-20, July, 1978.)

ery of health services on a continuum. The continuum involves the delivery of services within the community (such as ambulatory care settings, neighborhood health centers, private practices, and home health agencies) and between the community and institutions (such as hospitals and nursing homes). "In 1976 over 36 million patients were discharged from short stay hospitals across the United States. This is an increase of three and one-half million from five years previous."[2]

Numerous studies point out the benefits of effective discharge planning for specific types of patient populations.* With the increase of monies spent on health care and the increase of patient discharges, health care providers and consumers must hold themselves accountable to planning for discharge.

The proportion of the gross national product (GNP) spent on health care in the United States makes this nation one of the largest spenders on health care in the world. In Fig. 1-1 is shown the dramatic increase in billions of dollars spent on health care from 1950 to 1977. One factor that augmented the GNP was the increase in expenditures for nursing home care. "From 1966 to 1975 nursing home expenditures rose more than 500 percent. Nursing homes account for 67 percent of the catastrophic institutionalized population and 50 percent of the national catastrophic costs."[2] Escalating costs in health care have stimulated governmental agencies to closely monitor monies spent in delivery of health care services. This money monitoring is being manifested in regulations that strictly govern expenditures.

*References 3, 5, 7, 9, 14, 16, 17.

The impact of national and local legislation on health care and in particular on discharge planning is so crucial that we have devoted an entire section to it in Appendix B.

Since many variables are involved in the costs of health care, it is difficult to isolate and measure the impact of discharge planning on these costs. Despite the absence of precise measurements, experience has revealed to many health providers that planning for discharge with patients has a great potential for cost effectiveness.[3,4,18]

Consideration for continuity of care and cost effectiveness has led to a rapid increase in the development of discharge planning programs within institutions across the country. In 1971 the first formal regulations governing discharge planning in acute care hospitals were passed in the state of Massachusetts (a copy of these regulations can be found in Appendix C). It is essential to note that these regulations stressed the importance of having public health nurses and social workers working together with patients and physicians in the discharge planning process. This new emphasis is not to negate the additional input of health providers from other disciplines. It simply points out that whereas, traditionally, discharge planning was exclusively in the area of social service, there is now recognition of the need for this responsibility to be disseminated among all health providers. No one individual possesses all the knowledge and expertise required to offer the comprehensive discharge plan that a patient deserves.

Although managerial practices in discharge planning will be discussed in detail later in this book, it is pertinent here to describe developing patterns in the eastern part of the United States. Generally, discharge planning departments in institutions are based in one of three areas: (1) within the nursing department, (2) within the social service department, or (3) as an independent department responsible to hospital administration. A recent survey of 27 facilities in the Greater Boston area showed that over 50% of the discharge planning departments are based within nursing departments.[1] This survey is discussed in Chapter 2, wherein hospital administration views the organizational placement of discharge programs.

There appear to be two major reasons for this shift in institutional locus of program responsibility from social service to nursing. First, the role of the social worker seems to be changing from interfacing patients with social systems, to creating therapeutic relationships with patients as a catalyst for the development of better coping patterns. Second, with the passage of Medicare legislation in 1965, payment for services received after discharge predominantly depended on the documentation of the "skilled nursing needs" of patients. This change caused many social workers to reach out to nurses to interpret the ever-changing definition of "skilled nursing care."

Since nursing is accountable for 24-hour patient care, it seems logical for the patient's primary or team nurse to coordinate discharge planning with the patient. This does not diminish the important role that social service consultants and members of various other disciplines play in the discharge planning process. It simply points out the strategic position nursing has with 24-hour patient responsibility.

It is difficult to state exactly where the discharge planning department should be placed in every institution. Obviously, nursing has an important coordination responsibility, regardless of where the department is located. Actually, the department should be placed where it can be most effective. To avoid territorial conflicts, and to strengthen the base of a discharge planning program, individuals from all major disciplines should be actively involved in creating and implementing the program. For more information on managing multidisciplinary territorial issues see Chapter 7.

TYPES OF EXISTENT DISCHARGE PLANNING PROGRAMS

There are two major types of discharge planning programs: direct service and consultation. In a *direct service program,* one person (or persons from several disciplines) works directly with the patient and family to carry out the specific activities of the discharge planning process. A *consultation program* involves a team of consultants from various disciplines who work closely with primary providers responsible for integrating discharge planning into their delivery of health care. The consultants are usually persons (such as community health nurses, social workers, dietitians, and physical therapists) educated and experienced in the area of discharge planning. They may be either full-time members of the discharge planning department, or contracted as liaisons from specific hospital departments or community agencies. For example, a dietitian may be contracted from the dietary department to act as a discharge planning consultant. With advancement toward the delivery of primary health care, the consultation type is gaining rapidly in popularity.

Consultation is a process that involves not only specific education for the person who plans to implement the role of consultant but also the education of primary providers in the appropriate utilization of consultants. The consultation type of program relies heavily on in-service education in discharge planning. So that primary providers are able to independently integrate discharge planning into their delivery of care, they must be continually informed regarding the current regulations and available community resources.

A discharge planning program does not necessarily involve direct service or consultation exclusively. Most programs have elements of both direct service and consultation, and the pendulum swings back and forth between the two areas during the operation of a program (Fig. 1-2). At times, for example, a consultant may need to act as a role model and provide direct service in discharge planning. It is important to point out here, however, that all too often persons from a discharge planning department tend to jump in and implement the discharge planning process themselves without setting a goal to transfer the process into the hands of a primary provider. Their eagerness may delay the development of primary provid-

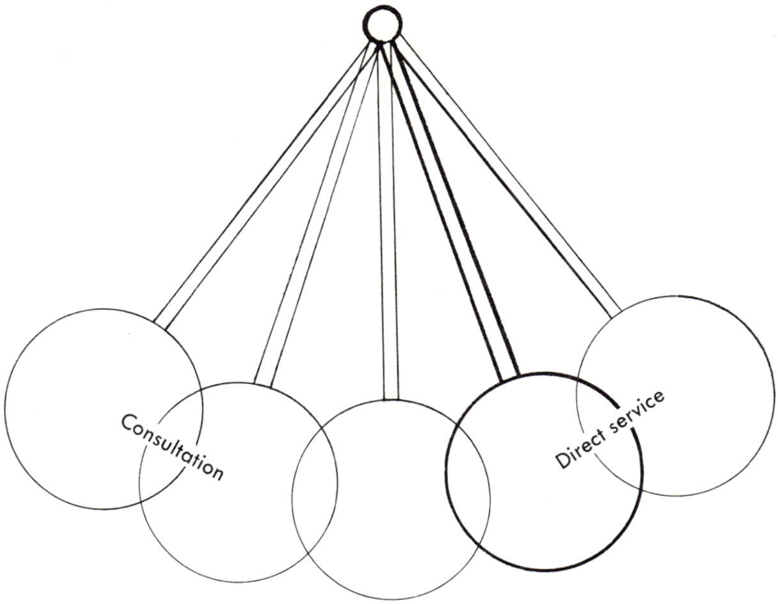

Fig. 1-2. Continuum of discharge planning.

ers toward more independent provision of care to patients. Furthermore, a direct service program usually requires a larger staff than a consultant program, and an increase in staff always results in an increase in budget.

SCOPE OF DISCHARGE PLANNING

The scope of discharge planning consists of four interacting elements: the patient and significant other persons, available resources, regulations, and primary providers of health care (Fig. 1-3). The focus of all these interactions is always the patient. *Patient participation in discharge planning is a cardinal principle*. Patients not only have the right to quality discharge planning but should, whenever possible, play the principal role of coordinating their own planning with the primary provider. Family members or significant other persons should be invited, with the patient's permission, to participate. Discharge planning should begin on the day of admission to allow ample time to complete an appropriate plan.

The second element in the scope of discharge planning is available resources, including the patient's home, the home of a significant other person, community agencies, and placement facilities. Approrpiate discharge planning cannot take place without adequate support systems outside the institution. Discharge planning consultants must be knowledgeable regarding the quality and quantity of resources and must impart this knowledge to primary providers. In many parts of the country, home health agencies are offering services up to 12 hours a day, with a proposed plan of increase to 24-hour coverage. This increased availability of both

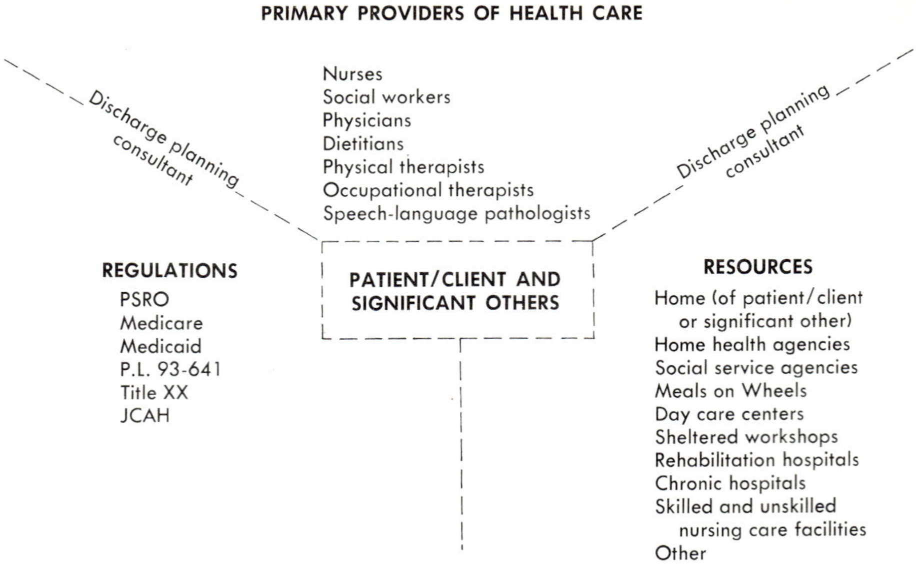

Fig. 1-3. Scope of discharge planning.

skilled and unskilled services has given more patients the option of home care as opposed to institutional care.

In communities where services are not available, it is important that continuing care consultants stand together to openly voice their concerns. Political pressure is a powerful force for change if utilized appropriately. For information regarding organizing an association of discharge planning consultants, refer to Chapter 4.

The body of regulations governing health care is the third element in the scope of discharge planning. Some regulations have helped to improve standards of care, and other regulations may have been responsible for setting up barriers to the achievement of qulaity. The important point to emphasize here is that discharge planning consultants must become more influential with the creators of regulations and more vocal in response to the effects of regulations. If we do not help to set the stage for discharge planning, it will be set for us, whether we approve or not. There are few things worse than living with a regulation that was created by someone whose ignorance in the area of discharge planning has caused many to suffer.

The fourth element in the scope of discharge planning is the responsibility of primary providers to integrate discharge planning into their delivery of health care. Institutions often tend to respond to "stressors" (such as new regulations) by isolating the stressed area and assigning a specific individual to perform the task that appears to solve the problem. I believe that even if there were one "discharge planner" for every patient, the process of discharge planning would be second-rate next to the integration of discharge planning within every health provider's deliv-

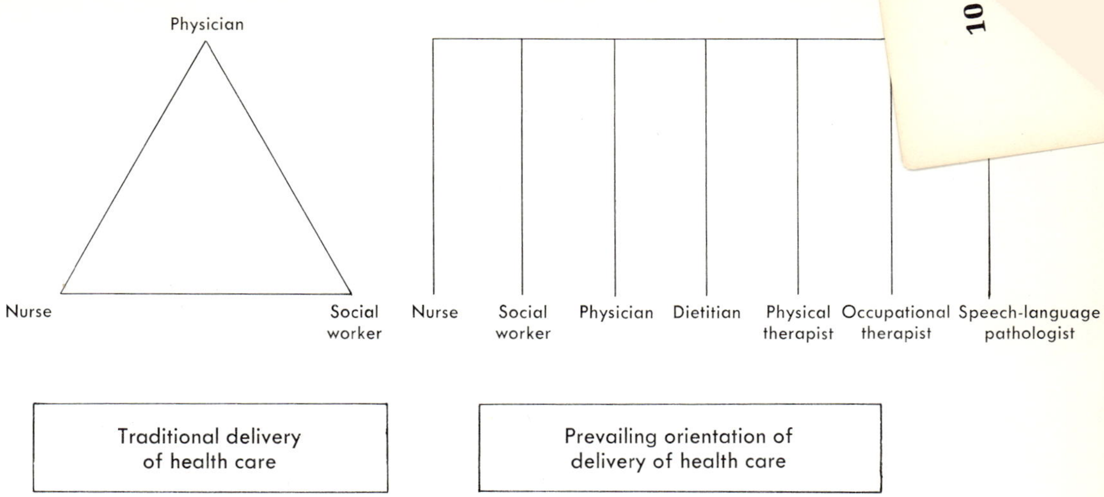

Fig. 1-4. Difference between the traditional approach to the delivery of health care and the currently prevailing orientation.

ery of care. To achieve this integration, persons from all health care disciplines should have available to them a "system" whereby they can carry out the discharge planning process with their patients. This system should be built on a threefold premise. First, individuals from all health care disciplines are equally accountable for their participation in discharge planning with patients. This equality can best be illustrated in Fig. 1-4, which shows the difference between the traditional approach to the delivery of health care and the currently prevailing orientation.

The second premise is that one primary provider should be designated joint coordinator of the discharge plan with the patient. This person should be the one who has greatest accessibility to the patient, family, and other health care providers.

The third premise is that a discharge planning consultant should be available to the primary care team members to provide them with current information and expertise that may enhance the discharge planning process.

DISCHARGE PLANNING PROCESS

Specific steps in the actual process of discharge planning parallel the five steps of problem solving shown in Fig. 1-5. They are (1) *assessment* of the patient's and family's present and prehospital patterns of life, (2) *diagnosis* of specific discharge problems based on the data gathered in the assessment, (3) *prescription* of plans to be carried out by the patient, family, and involved providers, (4) *implementation* of plans mutually chosen by the triad of patient, family, and health care providers, and (5) *evaluation* of the plans actually carried out.

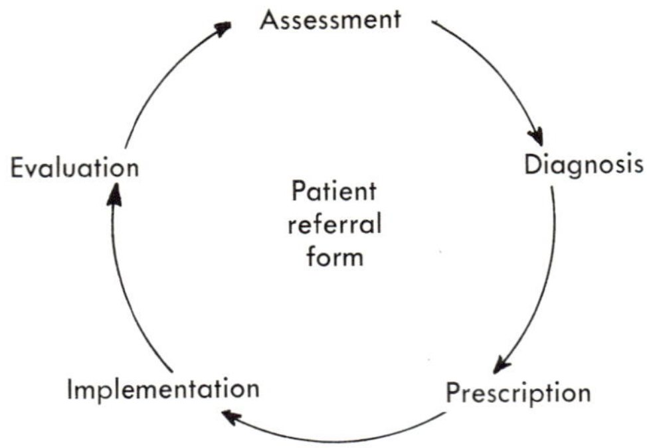

Fig. 1-5. Discharge planning process.

Referral form

If discharge planning is to achieve high standards of patient care, it will have to be supported by systematic documentation. This means that a uniform referral form, including all relevant information, should be used by all persons involved in the discharge planning process. Informal referring, consisting primarily of telephone calls or information loosely placed in writing, is usually inadequate and should not be ethically acceptable to health care providers. Many individuals in discharge planning are accustomed to the "open" method of referral forms, in which multiple disciplines simply document their problems and plans, utilizing their own terminology. This type of open referral is often more discipline oriented than patient oriented. It also lends itself to misinterpretations, because some disciplines utilize a taxonomy not understood by other disciplines. A referral system utilizing a uniform assessment terminology is essential for the transfer of information from one health care provider to another. Such a system will then be a factor in promoting continuity of care for the patient.

There are three major patient populations encompassed in most health systems: adult, pediatric, and maternity. Based on the fact that these three populations usually have different health problems that may require different responses from the support system in the community, the classification of assessment information and needs may differ slightly for each population. Some classifications, however, may cut across patient populations. For example, Katz and associates[8,9] developed an index of activities of daily living (ADL) that has been used for children as well as adults, mentally retarded as well as physically disabled persons, and noninstitutionalized as well as institutionalized persons. Their research has shown that ADL function tends to be lost and regained in a hierrarchical order, which makes it possible to rank the overall functional status of persons in a highly organized manner over time. *Discharge planning personnel must continue to be aware of nationwide work being done in the area of standardized patient care referral forms if they truly intend to affect the quality of health care delivered to their patients.*

It is beyond the scope of this chapter to discuss in detail all the research that has been done on standardized referral forms over the past 20 years. The reader is encouraged to refer to the annotated bibliography in Appendix A, where articles related to referral form research and construction are marked with an asterisk.

This chapter will present a summary of selected research, followed by specific issues that relate to the prupose, characteristics, and content of a referral form.

Selected research on referral forms. The Commission on Chronic Illness in the United States was created in 1949 and continued to function until 1956. One of its recommendations was for development of a taxonomy for use in evaluating patients for appropriate treatment and to provide a means for more economic use of available resources. From 1965 to 1969 the Public Health Service sponsored a series of workshops that focused on developing a *uniform system* of patient assessment.[15] The results of the workshops did not yield a particular product; however, participants were encouraged to continue experiemntal programs in various settings. As a direct outgrowth of these deliberations, a patient assessment system was developed by four research groups in 1973.[6] In 1978 Jones and associates[5] reported that they had utilized the patient assessment system developed in 1973 and had successfully tested it in several nursing homes and a chronic disease hospital in Boston. On June 21, 1974, the Department of Health, Education, and Welfare announced a campaign to upgrade the quality of care provided in the nation's nursing homes. One feature of this campaign was the use of a standardized patient assessment form called PACE (patient appraisal, care planning, and evaluation), which reflected current field experience with various assessment forms. The PACE tool was published in 1978 in a book entitled *Working Document on Patient Care Management: Theory to Practice*.[19]

Purpose of referral form. The purpose of a referral form is to provide a reliable method for the transfer of patient information from one health care provider to another. The referral form should contain two major components of information: (1) objective patient assessment and (2) care plans designed to meet the needs determined by the assessment. Ideally the form should also provide space for reevaluation and replanning by the receiving agency. A formal written referral is the primary rational basis for communication in the discharge planning process. Because of periodic mail loss and delays in mail delivery, verbal communication is encouraged as a supplement to ensure that the written information reaches its destination.

Characteristics of referral form. According to Jones and associates[6] and the Division of Long-Term Care of the Department of Health, Education, and Welfare,[19] each of the two components of information in the referral from previously mentioned should have the following characteristics: The patient assessment component should be *patient oriented,* describing the person as he is at the time of assessment; *multidimensional,* providing information from several perspectives (physical function, impairments, medical risk factors, and sociodemographic status); *objective* rather than subjective; and *relevant* to the purposes for which the assessment was intended. The care planning component, in addition to suggested plans, should provide space on the form for a reevaluation of the patient's discharge problems and should propose a time for reappraisal.

Content of referral form. The content of a referral form should directly relate to its purpose; therefore content items should include components of patient assessment, care planning, and space for evaluation at the receiving agency. A working panel of the National Center for Health Statistics (DHEW) has constructed a Minimum Data Set regarding information that should be included on referral forms for long-term care.[11] This list is useful as a starting point for the construction of a referral form for various patient populations.

All the research previously noted and some of the articles in the annotated bibliography (Appendix A) that are marked with an asterisk offer excellent examples of specific categories of content for referral forms. I strongly encourage anyone constructing a referral form to try to utilize categories of content that have been successfully tested. Patient care often suffers because time is wasted when one starts the monumental task of constructing a referral form from scratch. It is important to emphasize here that, if possible, the same referral form should be used to refer patients for home health care as well as for facility placement.

Discharge planning implementation model

The discharge planning implementation model proposed in this chapter is a model that represents the interaction between teams of individuals from several disciplines and the functions they perform in the process of discharge planning (Fig. 1-6).

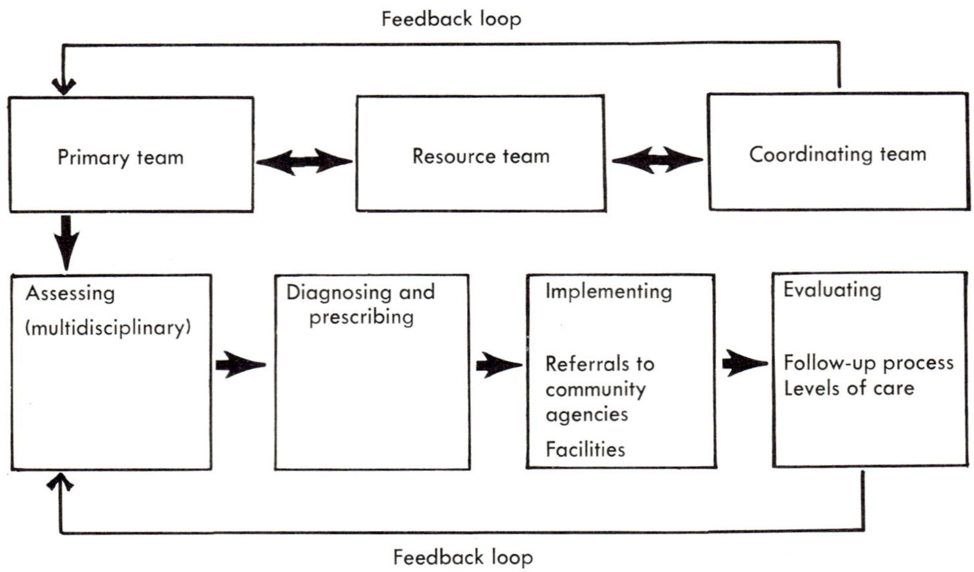

Fig. 1-6. Discharge planning implementation model.

Implementation of discharge planning begins with the *primary team,* which consists of the persons directly responsible for the care of the patient on a day-to-day basis (such as nurses, social workers, physicians, dietitians, and physical therapists). Their functions include the steps of the discharge planning process: *assessment,* data collection that relates to the patient's status at the time of discharge; *diagnosis,* statement of problems related to discharge; *prescription,* plans to meet the specific problems; *implementation,* actual writing of referrals to community agencies; and *evaluation,* following up with the community resource and the patient regarding the effectiveness of the discharge plan. To achieve the goal of a collective discharge plan, each professional provider is responsible for communicating with other providers and with the patient. If numerous providers are involved, it is helpful to have a predischarge planning meeting that, in addition to providers, includes, when possible, the patient, family, and representatives from the community agency.

The resource team and the coordinating team compose the next sections of the discharge planning implementation model. The difference between these two teams lies primarily in their distinct focus. The resource team is involved in consultation regarding the discharge problems of patients currently in the hospital. The coordinating team is involved in consultation regarding the problems of patients outside the hospital setting. An explanation of the composition of both teams and a delineation of their roles might further illustrate their differences.

The *resource team* includes a community health nurse (from the hospital's discharge planning program or from a community agency or both) and representatives from social service, medicine, and any other appropriate disciplines. Their role is threefold: (1) to be present at a specified time each week on all units to meet with the nursing personnel regarding current discharge problems (this activity is often referred to as rounds*); (2) to be available for emergency problems involving discharge (this availability is enhanced with the use of a beeper); and (3) to evaluate specific community resources such as home care services, chronic disease hospitals, and nursing homes.

The *coordinating team* includes the community health nurse from the discharge planning program and consultants from appropriate disciplines and specialty areas such as hospital administration and ambulatory care. Their role is to evaluate with primary providers the ongoing plan of care of outpatients with multiple complex problems. This team meets on a regular basis. It is helpful to invite representatives from the community agency serving the patient, since they can provide added information on the patient's current status and care plan. The role of the coordinating team does *not* replace or duplicate the role of the primary providers, but offers an adjunct service of consultation. The functions of the team members do not extend beyond the capacity to "advise." The primary responsibility of patient

---

*For more information on rounds, see Chapter 7.

care still rests with the primary providers. Factors affecting the success of multidisciplinary team meetings are discussed in Chapter 7.

Follow-up is the only way to evaluate the status of patients and validate the team's discharge plans. The simplest mechanism for follow-up is the enclosure of a follow-up form with all referrals, to be mailed back to the referring institution within a specified period of time. It is important to have all follow-up sheets mailed to one place, usually to the discharge planning department. Enclosing a stamped, self-addressed envelope helps ensure the reliability of return. A copy of the sheet can be sent to the primary team members who were involved with the patient. An alternative to sending a follow-up sheet with *all* referrals is to randomly select referrals for direct follow-up at some specified time interval after discharge. It is important, however, that a large-enough sample be selected for statistically significant results.

A useful basis for scheduling follow-up reviews or conferences derives from the concept of *levels of care*. In 1974 the National League for Nursing (NLN) sponsored a workshop on patient discharge and referral planning and published the proceedings.[12] The NLN workshop publication stated that, at a national level, home health services are being described as intensive, intermediate, and maintenance services. This classification provides an excellent structure for assigning a level of care to patients who have been referred to both nursing homes and home health agencies. The purpose of assigning a level of care is to group patients according to intensity of service needs so that follow-up evaluations can be made in timely fashion. Conferences are held more frequently on patients with higher levels of care. Inviting representatives from the community agencies to follow-up conferences provides a means of support to providers who are often isolated in the community.

An *advisory committee* is an important component in the discharge planning implementation model. If the members are carefully selected, they can provide that necessary link between the facility and the community which is so essential in delivering quality patient care.[13] The composition of an advisory committee should include representation from both the institution and the community. For example, representation from the institution could include the following: director of the discharge planning department, director of the nursing department, director of social service, director of medicine, director of dietary department, director within the hospital administration, and so on. If a director cannot attend the meetings, a delegate could be sent, as long as the same delegate is consistently present at all meetings. Community representation usually includes administrative representatives from various disciplines in community agencies (e.g., home health agencies, social service agencies, and neighborhood health centers). It is important to include consumers on the advisory committee. They provide an excellent feedback mechanism that is valuable in ongoing program development.

Advisory committees are often an extension of the planning committee, which had the primary responsibility of creating the discharge planning program. One of the major problems of an advisory committee is a lack of understanding among its members regarding their role. For example, to have the committee rubber-stamp the progress of the program is poor utilization of time and effort. Committee members need to believe that they are a vital force in the implementation of the discharge planning program. One creative way to utilize an advisory committee is to engage the members in carrying out a program audit, allowing them the opportunity to see the program in operation. (Program audits are discussed in Chapter 5.)

The discharge planning implementation model described in this chapter has been successfully implemented for more than seven years in an acute hospital setting.[10] It is assumed that this system is applicable to general or specialty acute hospitals, chronic disease hospitals, and nursing homes. The system should be modified to meet the specific needs of patients and the institution.

Outcomes from the implementation of this model have been numerous. They include (1) the provision of a framework to integrate discharge planning into every primary provider's delivery of care, (2) the enhancement of multidisciplinary team communications, (3) a linkage between the institution and community resources, (4) the creation of a format for evaluating discharge plans of patients, and (5) the provision of a mechanism for professional accountability to discharge planning. Interrelating the steps of the discharge planning process enhances the accomplishment of quality patient care. The discharge planning implementation model offers a framework in which that interrelationship could take place.

PROCESS OF CHANGE AND DISCHARGE PLANNING

Change is not easy and it takes time. For this reason it is important that discharge planning personnel have a working knowledge of the change theory. Institutions, particularly acute care hospitals, are usually crisis oriented. Therefore providers within hospital settings are not accustomed to being accountable to patients after discharge. Regulations, as well as patients themselves, are forcing institutions to extend their responsibility from crisis intervention to disease prevention and health promotion. This change is bringing about an added responsibility for individuals from various disciplines to incorporate discharge planning into their delivery of care. Because tighter budgets often cause diminished staffing patterns, the added responsibility of discharge planning may be met with some resistance both by primary providers and hospital administrators. Individuals may prefer familiar problems to unfamiliar solutions. Some institutions have attempted to meet problems regarding discharge planning in the traditional task-oriented fashion, assigning an individual to do the planning. As mentioned before, this is usually a second-rate approach to integrating discharge planning into the care delivered by primary providers. No one person can be a specialist in discharge planning *and* in medicine, nursing, social service, nutrition, physical therapy, occupational therapy, and speech-language pathology. Primary providers need a discharge planning consultant to keep them abreast of regulations and available community resources. However, the actual integration of discharge planning can best be accomplished within the various disciplines.

SUMMARY

In summation, discharge planning is a current priority in the delivery of health care services. The conceptual framework proposed in this chapter consists of three components: the scope of discharge planning, the process of discharge planning, and a discharge planning implementation model. These three components are intended to cover the *domain* of discharge planning, the *structure* of discharge planning, and a *format* for implementing a formal program in discharge planning.

Patient participation in discharge planning is a cardinal principle. Persons from various disciplines have a distinct responsibility in discharge planning with their patients. If possible, patients should coordinate their own discharge plans with a delegated primary provider. Since the discipline of nursing is accountable for 24-hour patient care and is in frequent contact with multiple health care providers, it appears appropriate in most situations that a member of this discipline be delegated joint coordinator with the patient. A discharge planning consultant should be available to primary health care providers. To avoid multidisciplinary territorial conflicts, persons from major disciplines must be actively involved in creating and implementing the discharge planning program.

REFERENCES

1. Greater Boston Continuing Care Coordinators—Resource Committee: Manual of continuing care departments in the Greater Boston Area. Unpublished manuscript, 1977.
2. Health, United States, pub. no. (PHS) 78-1232, Hyattsville, Md., Dec. 1978, Department of Health Education, and Welfare, p. 307.
3. Hoff, B., Johnson, J., and Williams, T.: A psychiatric assessment unit for readmission screening in a VA hospital, Hosp. Community Psychiatry **28**:177, March, 1977.
4. Izsak, F., Engle, J., and Medalie, J.: Comprehensive rehabilitation of the patient with cancer: five-year experience of a home-care unit, J. Chronic Dis. **26**:363, 1973.
5. Jones, E., Densen, P., and McNitt, B.: Assessing the quality of long-term care, 78-3192, Washington, D.C., 1978, Department of Health, Education, and Welfare.
6. Jones, E., McNitt, B., and McKnight, E.: Patient classification for long-term care: user's manual, pub. no. 74-3107, Washington, D.C. 1973, Department of Health, Education, and Welfare.
7. Juntti, J. J.: Problem solving in arranging for comprehensive home care, Nurs. Forum **8**:103, 1966.
8. Katz, S., and Akpom, A.: A measure of primary sociobiological functions, Int. J. Health Serv. **6**:493, 1976.
9. Katz, S., Ford, A., Down, T., and others: Effects of continued care: a study of chronic illness in the home, Pub. no. 73-3010, Washington, D.C., 1972, Department of Health, Education, and Welfare.
10. LaMontagne, M., and McKeehan, K.: Profile of a continuing care program emphasizing discharge planning, J. Nurs. Adm. **5**:22, 1975.

11. Long-term health care: minimum data set, Washington, D.C., 1978, National Center for Health Statistics, National Committee on Vital and Health Statistics, Department of Health, Education, and Welfare.
12. National League for Nursing: Patient discharge and referral planning—whose responsibility? pub. no. 20-1515, New York, 1974.
13. Oregon State Health Division, Community Health Nursing Section: Home health agency advisory committee reference guide, Portland, Ore., 1972.
14. Pryer, M., and Destagano, M. D. K.: Short-term follow-up evaluation of a rehabilitation program for multiple readmission psychiatric patients, J. Community Psychol. **1**:180, 1973.
15. Ryder, C., Elkin, W., and Doten, D.: Patient assessment, an essential tool in placement and planning of care, Health Rep. **86**:923, 1971.
16. Stephens, L.: Introducing a stroke service in a general hospital setting, Am. J. Occup. Ther. **29**:418, 1975.
17. Tolkoff-Rubin, N., Fisher, S., O'Brien, J., and Rubin, R.: Coordinated home care: the Massachusetts General Hospital experience, Med. Care **16**:453, 1978.
18. White, J.: Effective discharge planning can help reduce hospital costs, Utah Nurs. **23**:24, Summer, 1972.
19. Working document on patient care management: theory to practice, pub. no. HSQB 78-010, Washington, D.C., 1978, Division of Long-Term Care, Health Standards and Quality Bureau, Health Care Financing Administration, Department of Health, Education, and Welfare.

ADDITIONAL READINGS

Abdella, F., Forest, H., and Chow, R.: PACE: an approach to improving the care of the elderly, Am. J. Nurs. **79**:1109, 1979.

Bristow, O., Stickney, C., and Thompson, S.: Discharge planning for continuity of care, pub. no. 21-1604, New York, 1976, National League for Nursing.

Chamberlain, J.: The use of a consultant in team development, J. Continuing Educ. Nurs. **5**:25, 1976.

Nursing Development Conference Group: Concept formalization in nursing, Boston, 1973, Little, Brown and Co.

Schein, E. H.: The mechanisms of change. In Bennis, W., Benne, K., and Chin, R., editors: The planning of change, ed. 2, New York, 1961, Holt, Rinehart and Winston.

Sedgwick, R.: The role of the process consultant, Nurs. Outlook **12**:773, 1973.

Steffl, B., and Eide, I.: Discharge planning handbook, New Jersey, 1978, Charles B. Slack.

CHAPTER 2

Hospital administration views discharge planning

MARGARET E. LaMONTAGNE
ROBERT D. EMERMAN

WHY A DISCHARGE PLANNING PROGRAM

When any program is proposed in a hospital, an administrator must consider a multitude of issues. Examples of these issues include the involvement of pertinent departments and obtaining commitments from individuals to the goals of the program. As a part of this consideration, the administrator should understand the underlying pressures and motivation for implementation of the program.

In the first part of this chapter, we will attempt to highlight many of the pressures and motivation that have a particular impact on the development of a discharge planning program. They include regulatory and reimbursement considerations as well as the outcomes of their application to the issue of comprehensive patient care.

Regulatory and reimbursement considerations

Recent trends in health care delivery have focused on discharge planning activities. One such trend is the growing realization that to be effective a health care provider must consider the total patient and therefore must organize programs so as to ensure coordination of services to that patient. The organization of a discharge planning program as it relates to comprehensive patient care will be discussed later. A second trend, the phenomenal growth in health care costs in the last decade and the increasing proportion of these costs borne by governmental agencies, has led to the promulgation of regulations designed to reduce costs, eliminate duplication, and, at the same time, ensure that patient needs are being met.

External regulations often help to set priorities in program development. The following discussion will deal with the hospital administration's view of regulations affecting discharge planning. These regulations are derived from state licensing agencies, the Joint Commission for Accreditation of Hospitals, Medicare and Medicaid legislation, and private, third-party insurers, as well as from professional standards review organizations (PSROs). (Further discussion of these regulations may be found in Appendix B.)

State licensure. In an attempt to address both comprehensive patient care and cost issues, some states, including the Commonwealth of Massachusetts, have promulgated regulations regarding discharge planning in hospitals. A copy of the regulations can be found in Appendix C. The Massachusetts regulations, as an addition to its "Licensure Rules and Regulations for Hospitals," mandates a "multidisciplinary service to aid the attending physician and [the] patient in planning for continuing care upon discharge from the hospital."

The regulations stress three major points:

1. Development and operation of a written mechanism for early screening of patients to determine their needs for continuing care services
2. Utilization of a social worker and a public health nurse working together for continuity of patient care
3. Establishment of a uniform, statewide referral form to facilitate multidisciplinary communication about patients between the hospital and other institutions and agencies

Accreditation. The standards of the Joint Commission on Accreditation of Hospitals (JCAH), as expressed in the *Accreditation Manual for Hospitals,*[1] place a good deal of emphasis on the importance of discharge planning. Also, reference to the need for and requirements of such a program is found in several discussions.

The manual, in a discussion of the rights and responsibilities of patients, states that when a patient is transferred to another facility, the patient must have received a complete explanation of the need for the transfer and what alternatives exist. In addition, the patient may not be transferred unless the recipient facility has accepted the patient. The responsible practitioner or delegate should inform the patient of health care requirements that are necessary after discharge from the hospital. Effective compliance with these basic statements of rights requires a well-organized discharge planning program.

The JCAH nursing standards state that every patient should have a nursing care plan, initiated on admission, that includes a discharge plan as part of the long-term goal. It is suggested that medical and nursing staff establish active liaison with community facilities and agencies to assist in the patient's transition to another facility or to the patient's home.

The Quality of Professional Services Standards is more specific regarding utilization review. Utilization review plans are to include a mechanism for provision of discharge planning that shall be started as early as a determination of the need for such activity can be made, so that discharge can be facilitated when an acute level of care is no longer required. Further, it is suggested that criteria for discharge planning be developed to identify patients whose medical, psychological, or social circumstances usually require discharge planning. In addition, nonphysician health care professionals should be permitted to initiate discharge activity as long as such situations are delineated in the utilization review plan. Discharge planning, in the context of this standard, is not limited to referral to long-term care facilities but encompasses a broad range of continuity of care after discharge from an acute care institution.

In the rehabilitation services section the JCAH manual, as in the nursing section, recommends that the treatment plan include a discharge plan created in coordination with the patient and family as well as with the referring physician and members of other disciplines.

Reference to discharge planning is also found throughout the social work services section. As a part of the requisites of an approved social work services program, staff must show evidence of appropriate training, education, and orientation in discharge planning issues. A key role of the social work services department is to work with the patient and family to adapt to the various modalities of appropriate postdischarge care and treatment.

The importance of JCAH accreditation cannot be overemphasized, and therefore the requirements of JCAH standards must be seriously considered and acted on. Clearly the broad emphasis placed on discharge planning throughout the JCAH standards provides the administrator with an effective tool in initiating such a program.

Reimbursement. Medicare and Medicaid legislation, through PSROs as well as Blue Cross, has established regulations that effectively tie reimbursement to hospital bed utilization. These regulations consequently exert pressure on hospitals to develop or increase their discharge planning services. Exceeding length-of-stay criteria as specified by the PSRO may result in loss of payment by third-party payers. Therefore the hospital must provide discharge planning to minimize the problems that can confront patients when they are faced with the termination of their third-party coverage.

The Medicare regulations originally promulgated in 1965 as Public Law 89-97 refer several times to discharge planning. Even though the Conditions of Participation for Nursing Standards does not specifically mention continuing care nor discharge planning, it does state that review and evaluation of nursing care and written nursing care plans are to be kept current daily. Since discharge planning should be an integral part of the delivery of care for all health providers, nursing is accountable to carry out and document the methods, approaches, and modifications of care necessary to ensure a quality discharge plan for the patient.

The social service section of the JCAH manual speaks more directly to discharge planning by stating that the social work department is to be included in planning for patient care so that the patient is able to make full use of inpatient, outpatient, or community extended care or home health services. Follow-up of discharged patients and cooperative activities with community agencies are listed as functions to be recorded. The Utilization Review Plan Condition of Participation states that review of the medical necessity for admission and duration of stay should take into account alternative use and availability of services and facilities outside the hospital.

As an example of a third-party insurer review plan, Blue Cross of Massachusetts requires a review of the necessity of inpatient services provided to its members. The review plan must meet the requirements of the PSRO having jurisdiction (for purposes of Titles V, XVIII, and XIX of the Social Security Act) for patients in the hospital's PSRO area. In addition, a number of diagnoses require early discharge planning monitoring because of the possibility of post-hospital rehabilitation needs. This monitoring requires discharge planning activity to begin earlier in the patient's stay than would be mandated elsewhere.

The PSRO program and its legislative impact are discussed in more detail in Appendix B. The evolution of PSROs has provided another incentive for hospitals to develop a discharge planning program to ensure that all steps are taken to effectuate the appropriate placement of a patient when it has been determined that the level of care required does not mandate a stay in an acute care facility. As will be seen later, however, such a determination is not always easily made, and numerous issues affecting patient care and reimbursement can arise.

Comprehensive patient care and cost considerations

Over the last decade the hospital has become the focal point in the provision of health care services. This development has increased demands on the hospital to coordinate services provided to patients both within and outside its walls. Cost containment pressures, as well as legitimate attempts on the part of the hospital to function appropriately as a key resource, have mandated the growth of discharge planning programs.

A discharge planning program can raise issues that go beyond the development of an appropriate discharge plan for a particular patient. These issues include reducing the total costs for many patients, pointing out the inadequacy of available services within the community, and even bringing to attention the fact that, for some patients, the discharge plan will mean an increase in cost because of improved need identification. For example, the transfer of a patient to a "less costly" facility or home does not always translate to an overall lower cost to that patient. Factors that must be taken into account in analyzing a particular situation and that might lead to an overall increase in length of stay or rehospitalization include the time required for the patient to adjust to a new setting and staff and, similarly, the need for assessment by and adjustment of this staff to the patient. If, in fact, the scope and quality of ancillary and support services in the receiving facility or community are not equal to what could be found in the acute care institution, it could take longer to accomplish goals and, at the same time, increase the risk of return to the original facility. In addition, the feelings of the patient and family regarding transfer must be considered. Although they are difficult to quantify, the emotional impact of transfer may be substantial and could lead to increased length of stay. Finally, the cost of the transfer itself must be figured into the equation.

Effective discharge planning and utilization review programs have often focused on the inadequacy of available services within the community. For example, a postoperative cancer patient undergoing radiation or chemotherapy treatment. This person does not live near the treatment facility and does not need to be hospitalized, but he does need a place to live and perhaps minimum 24-hour health supervision. Not only are such living arrangements difficult or impossible to find, but cost and payment mechanisms are problematic or nonexistent. At one time, such patients stayed in the acute care facility after surgery, and there was third-party reimbursement. Now, if a need for acute care cannot be defined, reimbursement may be denied. As laudatory as the efforts of review programs may be to improve bed utilization and decrease health care costs, the difficulty of providing living arrangements, much less supervised placement, and the lack of reimbursement create a hardship for patients and hospitals alike.

It is important to recognize that an effective discharge planning program can be in a position to assess the total needs of the patient and to be influential in working with regulators, reimbursers, physicians, administrators, and others to ensure that the appropriate use of a variety of resources is accomplished. What is needed is education regarding health care services, closer communication between regulatory and provider agencies, and the development of systems to facilitate the flow of patient care information among providers of health care. (Chapter 4 discusses the development of an association of discharge planning consultants.)

HOSPITAL ADMINISTRATOR'S ROLE IN DISCHARGE PLANNING PROGRAM

Administrators have an important role in planning, organizing, and implementing a discharge planning program. In the development of a new program, it is essential that there be a commitment throughout the organization. The success or failure of the program may well depend on the strength of this commitment. Administration must set the tone and provide leadership in the planning process. It must ensure that all appropriate departments are included; that communication among departments and with the medical staff is open and constructive; that program development deadlines are met; and that program development is consistent with general institutional goals and objectives. Administration is also responsible for selecting the leadership of the program and for placing the program appropriately within the hospital organization. It has almost become trite to talk about multidisciplinary team delivery of health care. However, this is the best approach to ensure that in the program definition all patient needs are considered and the many diverse services are well coordinated.

Identification of need

The initial step in planning a program should be the identification of need. As important as deciding that the program is needed is determining its magnitude. This step can best be accomplished from within the institution by persons familiar with the patient population. The information will lead to the development of a systematic approach to case finding and the identification of patient needs. A planning committee should assist in development of this methodology and then be assigned the responsibility of outlining the discharge planning program.

Program planning and communication

An essential aspect of the planning process is to set dates for the expected completion of the various steps in the development of the program. Setting time-limited goals not only forces completion of various phases of the program but also sets the stage for ongoing evaluation. In the appointment of the planning team, it is obviously necessary to include certain departmental representatives. It is also important, however, to ensure that all departments that will be, or may be, affected are represented.

The initial planning group should be composed of representatives of departments most directly involved with the provision of care. Usually these departments will include at least nursing, social service, and medicine. Staff assistance by hospital administration is crucial. Other departments that should be involved in the process, although not necessarily represented on the core committee, include dietary, pharmacy, physical therapy, occupation therapy, and speech-language pathology, among others. Since documentation of discharge planning services should be a part of the patient's record, and since prompt medical discharge summaries to facilitate transfer communications are usually mandatory (for example, within 72 hours after discharge in Massachusetts), the director of medical records should be included at some point during the planning. The emphasis placed on level of care assessment and discharge planning by utilization review and PSRO requirements would support inclusion of utilization review coordinators in the planning process as well.

The importance of an open communication process must be emphasized. Issues surrounding control of the program are bound to arise during the process of selecting the appropriate organizational approach. If the full involvement of various disciplines is ensured, and if an environment is created in which members of the disciplines can interact on an equal level, a greater understanding of the overall goals and objectives of the program will be realized.

Organizational placement

There are numerous organizational alternatives for discharge planning programs, as illustrated in Fig. 2-1. The program may be placed entirely within the nursing department (Fig. 2-1, *A*), or it may be placed entirely within the social service

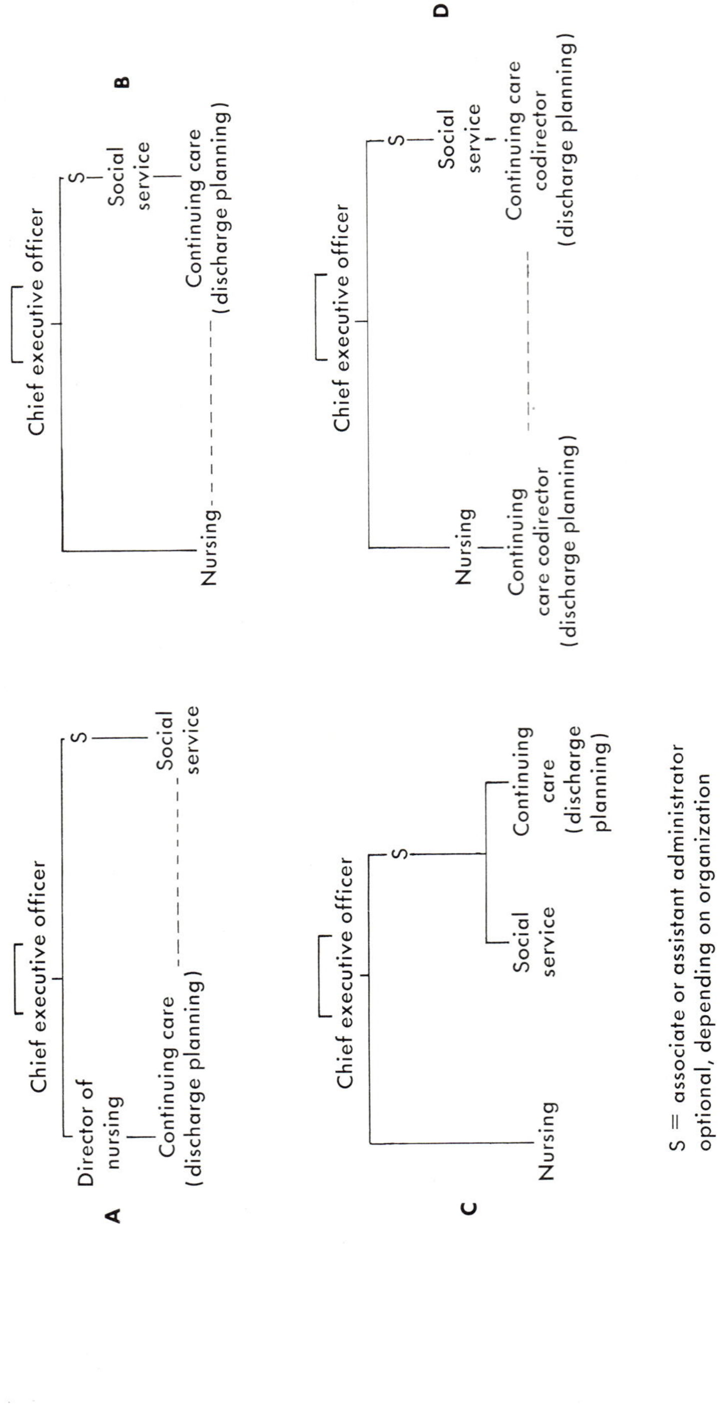

Fig. 2-1. Organizational alternatives for discharge planning programs.

department (Fig. 2-1, *B*). The director of the program might also report to an administrative officer who is neither a nurse nor a social worker (Fig. 2-1, *C*). Finally, the program could be co-directed by a nurse and a social worker, each of whom reports separately through the individual professional department (Fig. 2-1, *D*). Of the several alternatives that are available, the appropriate one will depend on various institutional considerations. A survey of 27 hospitals in the greater Boston area indicated that 48% of the programs surveyed were directed through the nursing department, and 16% were directed through the social service department. Twelve percent were coordinated jointly by the social service and nursing departments, and 24% received direction by an administrative officer who was neither the director of nursing nor the director of social service. Generally, except in unusual circumstances, the program should report administratively to one person to ensure that there is no confusion in role determination, in reporting relationships, or in location within the hospital structure. Because the program needs to be multidisciplinary in its approach, it is essential, regardless of the organizational placement, that the resources of nursing, social service, and other departments are tied into the system in a defined manner.

The discharge planning program primarily assists the patient in a smooth transition from hospital to home or to another facility. Many discharge planning programs have focused on facility transfers and referrals to community health nursing agencies. Consequently the necessity for identification of the need for skilled nursing care is important both from the point of view of patient care and in meeting reimbursement requirements. This emphasis has made placement of the program in the nursing department a logical approach. Nursing responsibility should ensure that communications between agencies regarding patient needs and nursing assessments are carried out by persons who are accountable for the 24-hour needs of the patient.

Discharge planning is obviously not limited, however, to facility transfer and community health nursing agency referrals. Many discharge plans require the coordination and provision of various nonnursing services, such as homemaking services, Meals on Wheels programs, physical and occupational therapy, and other supportive services. The ability to structure a multidisciplinary team, unit, or alliance, in a well-defined approach that is consistent with the overall goals and organization of the institution, is clearly essential to the success of any discharge planning program.

Allocation of resources

The administrative role in the planning process of a program also encompasses the allocation of such resources as space, staffing levels, and the hospital's dollar commitment to the program. Resource allocation should be made with the understanding that a discharge planning program will not take the place of another program or decrease social service or nursing positions. There will be additional expense to the institution initially, although the possible future savings in health care costs must be taken into account. As mentioned earlier, regulatory requirements mandate such a program, and the overall needs of the patient dictate its development. In fact, coordination of services to the patient may allow an institution to more effectively utilize its own resources.

It would be helpful to mention other economic issues that can be expected as early discharge planning becomes an integral part of the delivery of health care. Decreased length of stay, which diminishes occupancy, may result in a reduction of reimbursement and a pressure to eliminate some beds. Early discharge of convalescent patients releases beds for use by acute patients, and additional or better-prepared staff may be needed to care for the increase in acutely ill patients. Conversely, when there is great pressure for beds, discharge planning can lead to an increase in admissions and thereby improve reimbursement, since new admissions usually generate more revenue in the first few days of the hospital stay.

Education

The importance, for all departments, of an initial orientation and consistent, formal, ongoing education to the discharge planning program must be stressed, in spite of the fact that all pertinent departments have been included in the planning process. Although the emphasis on such education will probably be in nursing and social service, the other departments mentioned earlier should be included in the educational process both for new and old employees. There should also be at least a yearly update for primary departments and for all department heads.

It should be emphasized that a successful discharge planning program *must* have the support of the hospital's medical staff members. They need to understand the organization of the program, the services that it can help to coordinate, and the mechanism for their own interface with the program. Every member of the medical staff should receive pertinent information concerning the program and have the opportunity to discuss it in an open forum such as a medical staff meeting. Orientation for new medical staff members, and continuing education for others, should be carried out on a regular basis. The structure of the discharge planning program should be such that physicians can provide input not only through the planning phases but also as the program continues to develop. The direct involvement of physicians at various levels within the operation of the program is an important adjunct to the educational process. An example of their involvement was given in Chapter 1, in a discussion of the model of discharge planning implementation.

Evaluation

Realistically, no program can begin without a definition and without the determination of objectives, since these components set the parameters for persons implementing the program as well as for those affected by it. The importance of this definition and objective-setting process is not fully appreciated until it is time for evaluation. Initially, an evaluation should occur after six months and then continue on a yearly basis. Measurement of the objectives and statistics, as well as of the feelings and suggestions of staff from the hospital and community agencies, should be included.

The use of a computerized tool that can measure the effect of discharge planning on patient care would be one method of accomplishing evaluation. However, to our knowledge such a tool has not yet been effectively developed.

Advisory committee

An advisory committee for a discharge planning program is perhaps not mandatory but can be helpful and informative. The committee assists the discharge planning department in continually evaluating itself by providing an opportunity for the department staff to report activities and to identify major issues facing the program at regular meetings. It can also serve as an important forum for input of new ideas. Representatives should include hospital administrators, medical staff, nursing staff, and social service staff, as well as members of community nursing associations and other appropriate agencies or institutions, and consumers.

SUMMARY

In summation, we have drawn the information contained in this chapter from our experience in designing a successful discharge planning program and administering it for over seven years. Beyond the mandates of regulation requirements, a discharge planning program is an essential part of a comprehensive care effort. The development of an effective program requires the involvement of the hospital administrator, to ensure that the program has been well integrated into the hospital structure and that the appropriate mechanisms of multidisciplinary communication have been established both for implementation and ongoing evaluation.

REFERENCE

1. Accreditation manual for hospitals, 1979 edition, Chicago, 1978, Joint Commission for Accreditation of Hospitals.

ADDITIONAL READINGS

LaMontagne, M. E., and McKeehan, K. M.: Profile of a continuing care program emphasizing discharge planning, J. Nurs. Adm. **5**:22, 1975.

Medicare regulations, Chicago, 1972, Commerce Clearing House.

CHAPTER 3

Designing teaching strategies for education programs on discharge planning

BARBARA R. POLLACK
KATHLEEN M. McKEEHAN

This chapter is based on the premise that the goal of any discharge planning program should be to adequately educate primary care providers to apply the principles of discharge planning in their own delivery of health care. It is these providers who are responsible for direct patient care. Ironically, many practitioners have never received any formal training in planning teaching programs, although patient education and multidisciplinary sharing are major components of their role.

This chapter is designed for the individual with little, if any, formal orientation to educational theories. The chapter will present one example of a framework that can be used to develop effective in-service education programs and instructional materials. Four teaching techniques that can be integrated into the discharge planning in-service program, including the use of selected instructional media, will be described in detail.

Since discharge planning involves persons from numerous disciplines, it is important that these persons be involved in in-service education programs—both as participants and as educators in the overall process. More-intensive in-service programs should be presented to those persons who have the most responsibility for coordinating discharge planning. However, it is essential to plan appropriate education sessions for all hospital personnel. Even hospital administrators and unit management personnel, although not usually involved directly in patient care, need to become familiar with the philosophy and function of the institution's discharge planning program. This involvement is an important element in the overall success of implementing the discharge planning philosophy of the institution.

A question might arise regarding which department or person should be responsible for facilitating the discharge planning in-service program. Should it be the in-service education department, or the discharge planning department?

The answer to this question often depends on the individual institution. However, an important consideration is that whereas discharge planning consultants are often more knowledgeable about the content areas of discharge planning, in-service education personnel are more knowledgeable in the area of educational planning. A joint effort between the two groups should be fostered so that discharge planning becomes an integral part of patient care. Above all, an open avenue of communication should be established, leading to the common goal of educating primary care providers in the principles of discharge planning.

BUILDING THE FRAMEWORK

For the teaching-learning process to be successful during any particular in-service effort, the program should be properly designed and developed. One way to ensure success is to use a systematic approach when developing the plan.

A systematic approach offers a logical way to define, develop, and evaluate instructional methods and materials needed to accomplish the program's objectives.[6,9,10,11] Four major elements of the problem-solving method can be used as guidelines in planning an in-service education program. In Fig. 3-1 is an illustration of the anticipated flow and overall relationship of these elements to each other, including the following steps:

1. Assessment of learning needs
2. Development of learning objectives
3. Design or selection of methods and techniques used to achieve the objectives
4. Evaluation of the achievement of the objectives

Each of these elements is further discussed and illustrated below.

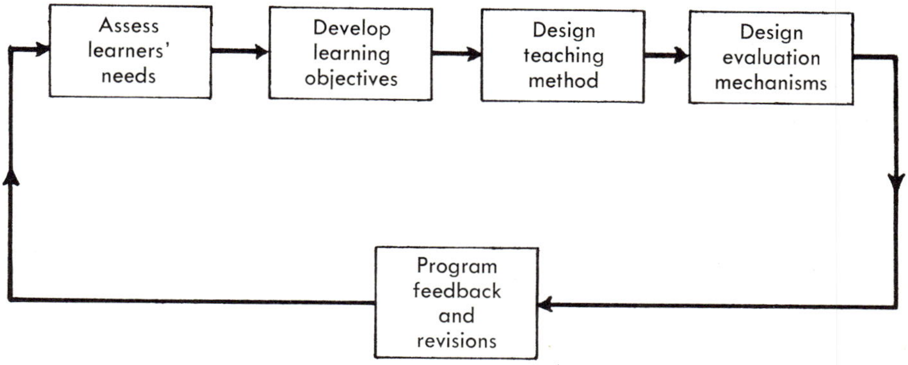

Fig. 3-1. Framework for systematically developing discharge planning in-service programs: four major elements of problem-solving method.

Step 1: Assessment of learning needs

Orientees come into hospitals today with a wide variety of skills and experiences. The first task in designing education programs is *to determine the entering learning behaviors of the participants* (Fig. 3-2). Are they familiar with the overall philosophy of discharge planning? Are they equipped with skills necessary to determine and assess a patient's discharge planning needs? Are they aware of existing community resources, of the levels of care available, and of the overall structure of the health care delivery system? Have they ever written interagency referrals?

It is crucial to know these previous knowledge levels and learning styles prior to the actual in-service program if the proposed plan is to be effective. After all, the ultimate goal of the in-service program is to teach members of the various disciplines what they do not know—not to reiterate areas in which they have already developed competence.

One way to gather this information is to present the participants with a pretest. A pretest will determine how much of what is to be learned during the in-service program is already known, will give the instructor the opportunity to modify the content, and will offer feedback to the learners concerning their expected attainment level.[6]

When designing a pretest, ask the question, What should the participants already know before beginning this in-service program? The results of the pretest will determine the overall content of the in-service program. For example, it might be established that as a prerequisite to the in-service program, participants must be able to identify community resources necessary for implementing discharge planning. After the pretest has been administered, it may be discovered that learners have not been able to meet this requirement. If the prediction of the learners' performance is to be realistic, the educational content of the program will have to be readjusted and reevaluated.

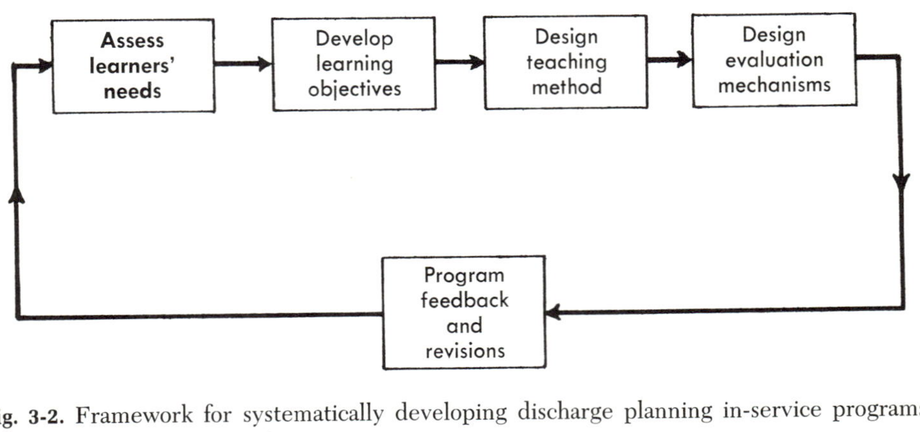

Fig. 3-2. Framework for systematically developing discharge planning in-service programs: assessment of learning needs.

During this planning stage, it is also essential to determine the structure of the learning environment. The following are essential questions: Will the learning take place in small-group or large-group settings, independent study sessions, or a combination of these methods? How much time will be available for the in-service education program? Who will be involved in the actual implementation of the program?

Step 2: Development of learning objectives

The next step in the development process is to determine effective goals and objectives (Fig. 3-3).

A goal is a broad statement of instructional intent.[6] In other words, it is what learners will know after completion of the in-service program. A goal for a discharge planning in-service program might be *to enable members of the various disciplines to effectively incorporate the principles and practices of the discharge planning process into their delivery of health care*.

Since learning indicates a change in behavior, a means of assessing the change should be established.[6] This is done by identifying and developing *behavioral learning objectives* that will enable the learner to reach the stated goal(s) of the discharge planning in-service program. For example, the following learning objective might be developed:

After listening to a lecture on "Regulations and Third-Party Payment Mechanisms and Their Relationship to the Discharge Planning Process," participants will be able to state, without error, the specific PSRO standards designated for discharge planning with patients.

It is the behavioral objective(s), not the overall in-service program goal, that assists the instructor in determining the most appropriate teaching strategy and in ultimately evaluating the entire teaching-learning process. Behavioral objectives will also provide the participant with the outcomes of instruction.

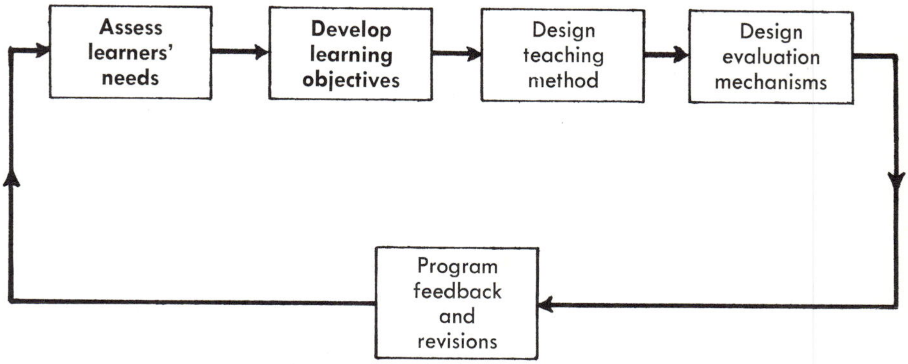

Fig. 3-3 Framework for systematically developing discharge planning in-service programs: development of learning objectives.

Behavioral objectives are classified under one of three main headings: cognitive, affective, and psychomotor.[3,6,15,17] Most in-service education programs are concerned with cognitive objectives, which describe information and knowledge. Affective objectives describe values, attitudes, emotions, and feelings. Psychomotor objectives. involve the manipulation of materials and objects and are ordinarily coordinated with cognitive learning.

Benjamin Bloom and associates[3,17] developed a classification, or taxonomy, of both cognitive and affective objectives that provides a basic framework for specifying human behavioral characteristics. The framework ranks the behavioral objectives according to the desired teaching-learning level. A taxonomy has not yet been developed for psychomotor objectives; however, Robert Kibler and co-workers[15] have formulated a set of subclassifications of psychomotor behaviors. Readers are encouraged to read the reference *Behavioral Objectives and Instruction*.

The Bloom taxonomies arrange cognitive and affective objectives into six major classes, reflecting an ascending level of competence for the learner:

	Cognitive	Affective
6.0	Evaluation	Characterization
5.0	Synthesis	Organization
4.0	Analysis	Conceptualization
3.0	Application	Valuing
2.0	Comprehension	Responding
1.0	Knowledge	Reading

The following is an example of a cognitive objective for discharge planning:

As a result of this in-service program, the participant will be able to correctly identify the members of the primary team and describe their relationship to the resource and coordinating teams.

The following is an example of an affective objective for discharge planning:

By the end of this in-service program, the participant will value working as a member of a multidisciplinary team in the discharge planning of a patient.

As a result of establishing these two taxonomies, an instructor can (1) plan programs around all learning levels, (2) make sure that instruction is provided to meet the prerequisite objective prior to attempting to teach complex objectives, and (3) ensure that appropriate evaluation instruments are employed to correspond with the stated objectives.[6] When the program's objectives are developed, not only are the lower-order objectives of knowledge, comprehension, and application utilized, but the learner's abilities to analyze, synthesize, and evaluate are tested.

For behavioral objectives to be useful in a learning experience, they must answer certain criteria. A good objective will answer the questions of who, what, when and how well. These characteristics are often called the ABCD format—audience (who), behavior (what), conditions (when), and degree (how well).[11] Action verbs such as to describe, to identify, to compare, and to contrast should be used in the body of the objective. These words are more readily measurable than vague words such as to understand or to know. For example, the discharge planning objective may state the following:

After being given a sample patient vignette focusing on the discharge planning process, the participant will be able to select at least four patient problems that would require intervention by the appropriate community resources.

The following ABCD components are present in the above objective:

Audience (who)	"the participant. . ."
Behavior (what)	"will be able to select. . ."
Conditions (when)	"after being given a sample patient vignette. . ."
Degree (how well)	"at least four patient problems. . ."

The following is another example of a discharge planning objective:

After viewing the slide-tape program on implementing the discharge planning process, the participant will be able to describe, without error, the procedures necessary for processing a referral to a community agency.

The ABCD components in the above objective are as follows:

Audience (who)	"the participant . . ."
Behavior (what)	"will be able to describe . . ."
Conditions (when)	"after viewing the slide/tape program . . ."
Degree (how well)	"without error . . ."

Many theories have been formulated on the use and development of behavioral learning objectives. The reader is referred to work by Kibler and associates.[15]

Step 3: Design or selection of methods or techniques used to achieve objectives

Once the established learning objectives are determined, the next step is the selection of an appropriate teaching method (Fig. 3-4). It is not uncommon to use

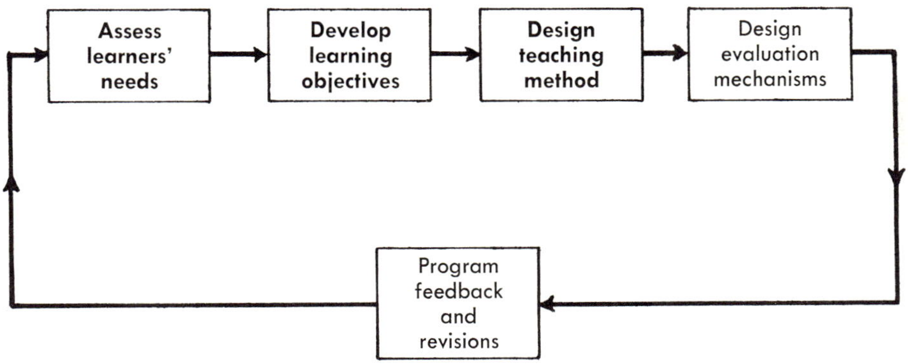

Fig. 3-4. Framework for systematically developing discharge planning in-service programs: selection of methods used to achieve objectives.

several different teaching techniques during an in-service education program. A different method or technique may be needed to reach the stated learning objective. Variables—including group size, allotted time for the in-service program, entering learning behaviors, motivation of the participants, and the way the information should be received, processed, and remembered—determine the teaching method that can be most effective. Current research findings indicate that there is more than one useful way to teach.[7]

Lectures, small-group discussions, demonstrations, instructional media, independent study, role playing, and patient studies are some of the teaching methods that can be used during in-service education programs. Four methods—lecture method, values clarification exercises, patient studies and instructional media techniques—that have proved successful in meeting established objectives for discharge planning in-service programs will be described in detail later in this chapter. Good references for all these teaching methods are Davis's *Teaching Strategies for the College Classroom*[7] and Barbour and Goldberg's *Interpersonal Communication: Teaching Strategies and Resources*.[1]

Step 4: Evaluation of achievement of objectives

The last step of the instructional process, as shown in Fig. 3-5, is evaluation. Evaluation is defined as "the continuous process of collecting and interpreting information to assess decisions made in designing and conducting instruction."[18] This step is often considered to be the *foundation* of the entire learning process. The information gathered during this step serves three purposes: (1) to provide the data for deciding whether the in-service program achieved its stated objectives; (2) to determine whether the teaching strategies and techniques were effective; and (3) to indicate the program's weak points so that revision can effectively occur.[13]

Instruction should be designed so that learners will be able to perform all tasks, ideally with complete success. It might be useful to assess learning several times

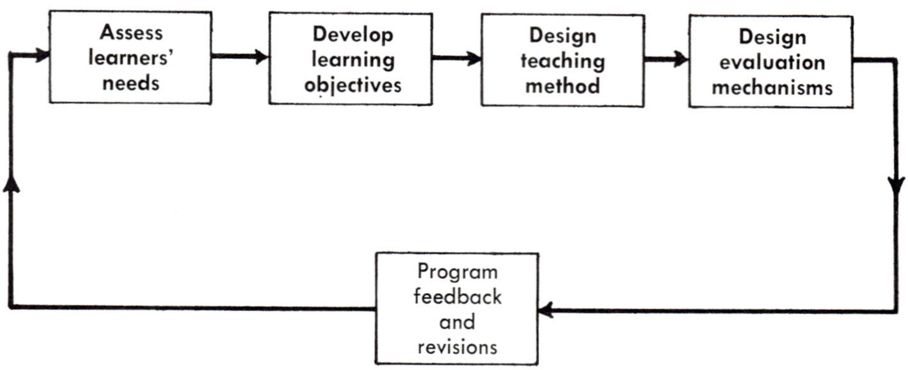

Fig. 3-5. Framework for systematically developing discharge planning in-service programs: evaluation.

during the in-service program. A written exercise is not necessary. Just asking participants verbally "where they are in comprehending the content" is adequate. If learners are not achieving the learning objectives, the in-service program should be modified. Administering a follow-up test immediately after the in-service program is advisable. The follow-up test can be the same as the pretest. If scores improve, learning has taken place.

It is also important to evaluate the participants' general opinions of the discharge planning in-service program. This can be done by developing *attitude scales,* in which the respondent is asked to circle a letter that indicates personal opinion on a five- to seven-point scale. The scale ranges between extremes such as agree-disagree or like-dislike.[12] An example follows:

1. After completing this discharge planning in-service program, I know I am more skillful in writing referrals to community agencies.

Strongly agree	Agree	Undecided	Disagree	Strongly disagree

The following is an example of another type of rating scale—the semantic differential—that measures attitudes using five to seven *polar adjectives* (adjectives opposite in meaning):

1. This discharge planning in-service program was

   Not useful 1 2 3 4 5 6 7 Useful

2. The multidisciplinary instructor was

   Boring 1 2 3 4 5 6 7 Dynamic

3. The in-service program was

   Disorganized 1 2 3 4 5 6 7 Organized

Participants rate the statements by placing an X somewhere along each of the seven-point scales according to their perceptions or feelings at the moment. The results are then graphed to obtain a profile.

Readers interested in more information on rating scales should refer to the work of Osgood and co-workers[19] on the measurement of meaning.

In addition to the participant's cognitive and affective evaluations of the discharge planning in-service program, it is important to ask participating instructors for their feedback. Questions such as, Were you comfortable with your teaching role? or Did you receive the necessary support to present your component effectively? will assist in ensuring the overall effectiveness of the in-service program. Equally important is the instructor's self-assessment of the in-service program: Were the learner's needs assessed adequately? Were the learning objectives too easy or too difficult? Were the teaching techniques exciting or boring?

The discharge planning in-service program should be evaluated in relation to the philosophical educational goals of the institution. For example, the philosophy of the nursing department might revolve around primary nursing care. The discharge planning in-service program could foster this philosophy by teaching nursing participants their specific role in incorporating discharge planning into their delivery of primary nursing care.

Analysis of the feedback (by both learner and instructor) may indicate a need to revise components of the in-service program. These revisions may range from minor to critical. The model depicted in Fig. 3-1 shows the instructional development process to be cyclical in nature. Therefore, if revision is indicated, start at step 1 (assessment of learning needs), and work through the remaining steps, making the appropriate changes before implementing the discharge planning in-service program again.

TEACHING METHODS FOR USE IN A DISCHARGE PLANNING IN-SERVICE PROGRAM

A sample content outline for a discharge planning in-service program is presented in Fig. 3-6. Both cognitive (acquisition of new knowledge) and affective (making decisions and determining actions) objectives are included in this in-service outline.

I. Philosophy of discharge planning within a particular institution.

II. Description of institution's discharge planning program/department, including:
   A. Definition
   B. Objectives
   C. Implementation methods
      1. Individuals responsible for coordinating discharge planning of patients
      2. Specific procedures for processing referrals

III. Legislation governing discharge planning, including:
   A. Federal legislation (Medicare)
   B. State legislation (Medicaid)
   C. Professional standards review organization (PSRO)
   D. Other

IV. Issues revolving around multidisciplinary communication

V. Available community resources

Fig. 3-6. Content outline for a discharge planning in-service program.

Learning involves content learning (acquisition of information) and process learning (the way the acquired information is used). *Content learning* is often referred to as the expository approach or passive learning.[2,9] The instructor presents the information, and the learners are expected to absorb and retain that information. *Process learning,* called the inquiry approach or active learning, involves learning through participation.[2,9] The instructor's role is to facilitate learning so that participants are able to raise questions and organize information. Both of these learning methods may overlap during an in-service education program. Lectures and instructional media techniques used during a discharge planning in-service program will achieve content learning; values clarification exercises and patient studies will achieve process learning.

Lecture method

The lecture is one of the most common teaching methods and is the most successful method in meeting lower-order cognitive objectives (knowledge, comprehension, application), particularly with large groups of learners. It is possible for lectures to achieve higher-order cognitive objectives (analysis, synthesis, evaluation) if new views and organizations of knowledge are being provided.[6]

Some content knowledge, such as information on current discharge planning legislation or an explanation of the steps in the discharge planning process, will need to be transmitted in a discharge planning in-service program. Lecturing is the method most often used to impart content knowledge. A lecture does not have to be mundane. It can be both enjoyable and effective if learner motivation and learning processes are taken into account. The use of the following techniques will tend to heighten audience interest during the lecture.

Begin the presentation by telling learners exactly why the topic deserves attention. Then identify key concepts to be covered during the lecture. The instructor should play an important role in helping learners to focus attention on the main ideas by encouraging feedback throughout the lecture. The use of *interactive lecture sheets* or *lecture summary sheets* will provide participants with a means of interacting with the learning environment.[20] These handouts not only offer learners an instant overview of the lecture but also minimize note taking, which hinders the actual learning process. For example, the lecture topic might be "Implementation of the Discharge Planning Process." Outline the main components of the lecture, as illustrated in Fig. 3-7, leaving enough space between the components so that participants can add the relevant information as the lecture progresses. The lecture summary sheet may contain diagrams and charts, as well as bibliography for further reading on discharge planning.

Overhead transparencies. Overhead transparencies are an excellent teaching tool to use during a lecture and will allow more time for questions and discussions. Overhead transparencies can be prepared simply and inexpensively. One of the most common materials used to make them is clear, uncoated acetate. Special felt-

Title: Implementation of discharge planning process

Directions: This summary sheet has been provided for you to immediately summarize the information that has been presented during this lecture. You may keep this sheet for future reference.

A. The five steps in the discharge planning process include:
   1.__________
   2.__________
   3.__________
   4.__________
   5.__________

B. The process fits into the following model:
   1. Primary team
      a. Assessment, multidisciplinary__________
      b. Patient diagnoses__________
      c. Referrals__________
      d. Levels of care__________
      e. Multidisciplinary team meetings__________
   2. Resource team
   3. Coordinating team
   4. Advisory team

C. Additional notes:

Fig. 3-7. Lecture summary sheet.

tip transparency pens, India ink, or china markers may be used to draw directly on the acetate.

Transparencies can also be made by mechanically reproducing prepared artwork. The most popular method, called the thermal process, uses a Thermofax machine, manufactured by the 3M Company. Any illustration made with a pencil, India ink, or a typewriter can be reproduced with a Thermofax machine. Colored, adhesive-backed films may be cut to shape and used for coloring large or small areas. Transparency film can be purchased that will show black lines against solid-color backgrounds or colored lines against a clear background.

Xerox machines can also be used to produce overhead transparencies. This is the most common way to produce transparencies; however, a special transparency film made exclusively for use on Xerox machines is needed. Overhead transparencies cost approximately 30 cents to $2 to produce. Overhead projectors cost approximately $200.

Values clarification exercises

Values clarification is an *intervention* method at helping individuals become aware of their current valuing system and learn how it might affect their attitudes, behavior, and decision making. Participants in a discharge planning in-service program bring with them personal, educational, and perhaps working experiences that affect their values. Values are sometimes altered when persons experience the shock derived from the differences between the educational world and professional practice in institutional settings.[16] This shock often manifests itself in feelings of powerlessness, fearfulness, apathy, and what is commonly termed "burnout." One of the causes of these feelings may be values confusion. The following example is an illustration of values confusion:

Patient study. A 90-year-old man and his family presented themselves to the emergency room staff of a large teaching hospital. The man's health history was known to the staff, and their assessment determined that the man was dying. A decision was made to take only palliative measures in treatment. Since hospital beds were limited that day, the physician decided to send the man back to the home of his family. A psychosocial assessment revealed a high level of anxiety in both the patient and his family, related to fear of the impending death. The following valuing issues may be confronting the persons involved in this situation:

- Which patients have the priority for hospital beds?
- Should the physician be permitted to have ultimate power to admit and discharge a patient?
- Should the emergency room team foster the discharge decision and enlist the help of a home health agency as a resource for the family, or is it up to the family to decide when outside help is needed?
- Should the emergency room team just accept the idea that their accountability to the patient has ended, and send the family home without concrete plans for follow-up?

Discharge planning can be integrated into the valuing process of the various disciplines only when individuals become aware of their own valuing in three areas: (1) their concept of discharge planning, (2) the use of community resources, and (3) their perceived role as an equal member in a multidisciplinary team.

The following strategies offer a few examples of how values clarification exercises can be used for discharge planning in-service programs. Because of time constraints, it may be possible to use only a few strategies during the in-service program. Brief objectives and suggested implementation methods are given for each exercise.

Strategy 1—Name tag

OBJECTIVE: To ensure a comfortable atmosphere conducive to the exchange of personal ideas

TIME NEEDED: 15 to 30 minutes for completing the name tag and additional time for group sharing

MATERIALS: Name cards and common pins

PROCESS

1. The objective of the activity is explained by the facilitator.
2. Participants are instructed to divide the name tag into four areas, with their name written in the middle of the tag.
3. Four questions (one at a time) are read by the facilitator. Participants write their responses sequentially in each quadrant of the name tag.
4. Participants are then divided into three or four small groups, where they share their responses with other group members.

Sample name tag questions

1. What do you enjoy doing with your leisure time?
2. List three things you would give to a significant other person if you were to die suddenly.
3. What kinds of qualities (your best assets) would you like your patients to see in you?
4. What kinds of qualities would you like your colleagues to see in you?
5. What adjectives best describe yourself?

Strategy 2—Sentence completion

OBJECTIVE: To stimulate participants to think about their role in the discharge planning process

TIME NEEDED: 3 to 5 minutes per sentence for writing answers; 45 minutes for the total activity, including discussion of answers

MATERIALS: Pencil and paper for participants

PROCESS

1. The facilitator reads several open-ended statements.
2. Participants complete the statements and then divide into small groups to share their responses. They may remain as a large group if desired.

Sample sentence completion questions

1. Discharge planning should begin when . . .
2. The most significant persons to be included in the discharge planning process are . . .
3. Past experiences with discharge planning taught me that . . .
4. The discipline that is usually responsible for coordinating discharge planning with the patient is . . .

It is important to emphasize that this strategy should be utilized in the beginning of the in-service program, to tap the preexisting values of the participant.

Strategy 3—Valuing questions

OBJECTIVE: To help participants define their role in the discharge planning process

TIME NEEDED: 30 minutes

MATERIALS: Pencil and paper for participants

PROCESS

1. The facilitator presents a patient study and asks participants to respond to a series of valuing questions.
2. The facilitator stresses that there are no "right" or "wrong" answers.

Sample patient study and valuing questions

PATIENT STUDY

NAME: Janet S.

AGE: 70 years old

FAMILY/ENVIRONMENTAL STATUS: widowed, with one child (son who lives 1 mile away); resides in four-room apartment, ground floor

MEDICAL DIAGNOSIS: cancer of the right breast (right modified radical mastectomy performed during this admission): S/P congestive heart failure; arthritis

PROFILE OF HOSPITAL STAY: Ms. S. was initially very frightened regarding her surgery and hospital stay. She gradually relaxed and related well to the staff and the support they gave her. The hospital stay reduced her mobility and caused secondary complications. Whereas she had previously used a cane to help her walk, she is now dependent on a walker. Presently her wound has a small amount of serous drainage, requiring a daily dressing change. This morning her physician tells you that Ms. S. will be discharged today. You begin to explore alternatives with the physician for discharge planning. As one alternative you recommend that a visiting nurse see her for dressing changes and an evaluation of her functional ability in the home. The physician replies that she has a supportive family and that filling out extra pieces of paper for the referral would require too much time.

VALUING QUESTIONS

1. How would you respond to the physician's response?
2. If the staffing had been short on your unit that day, what would your priorities for nursing care have been for this patient on her day of discharge?
3. Would your values be the same if you had had more time?

Readers are encouraged to develop their own values clarification exercises and are referred to the work by Diane Uustal.[22,23]

Patient study method

This teaching technique provides an excellent opportunity for participants to engage in actually implementing *all* the steps of the discharge planning process.

For example, based on a profile of a patient's hospital stay, participants can

- Assess the patient's current condition and projected discharge status
- Diagnose possible discharge problems
- Create a tentative plan to meet the problem
- Implement the plan by actually writing a hypothetical referral
- Evaluate the plan by suggesting follow-up methods

The instructor can create the patient studies, or the participants might go to units and write referrals on patients who have actual discharge problems. It is important to emphasize here that if actual patients are utilized, staff support will be needed due to the participants' lack of experience. Sometimes it is helpful to have small groups of participants work on the same patient study.

Once the referral is written, each participant or group of participants presents the referral to the other group members. An opportunity is thus provided for exposure to a variety of patients with discharge problems.

Instructional media techniques

An array of audiovisual instructional materials can be utilized during in-service education programs. Audiovisuals are ideal for solving recurring training problems, such as the need to repeat in-service sessions due to frequent staff turnover, or to train all three nursing shifts as well as persons from multiple disciplines. Use of overhead transparencies, as previously discussed, audiocassettes, slides, or a combination of slides and audio will effectively and efficiently facilitate discharge planning in-service programs. Readers who wish more information on the characteristics and preparation of other audiovisual media are encouraged to refer to the publication of Brown and co-workers entitled *AV Instruction: Technology, Media, and Methods*,[4] and to Bullough's *Creating Instructional Materials*.[5]

Audiocassettes. Audiocassettes are among the least expensive, most readily available, and most versatile of learning resources. Audio recording itself is simple, and the equipment is easy to operate. Audiocassette recorders average in cost from $50 to $150, and cassette tapes cost from $1 to $5.

Audiocassettes are excellent for preserving live discussions containing pertinent information, such as a discussion with community health nurses concerning their experiences while working with dying patients and their families. Audiocassettes and recorders are ideal for mobile in-service programs. Movable equipment carts can be stacked with audiocassettes on a variety of topics and then wheeled from unit to unit during various shifts. This process enables learning to take place in a self-paced, self-controlled, and self-contained environment.

Education research has shown that approximately 83% of what we learn is through the sense of sight, and that when a *combination of audio and visual media* is used, the result is significantly higher than when either medium is used alone. More learning results when the visual message complements and supplements the verbal message, rather than merely repeating it.[24] Although production is time consuming, a combination of slides and audiocassette is worth the effort. This process facilitates better organization and condensation of information, as well as a more efficient presentation. A lecture that normally requires one hour to present can be reduced to 15 minutes.

Slide-tape presentations. Slide-tape presentations usually comprise two or three components—an audiocassette, 35 mm slides, and a summary sheet or response booklet.[21] The audiocassette is the major source of information and controls the learner's interaction with the slides. The slides enrich the narration by providing examples. The response booklet or summary sheet provides an outline for review and reference. The entire system can be used for individual or group learning.

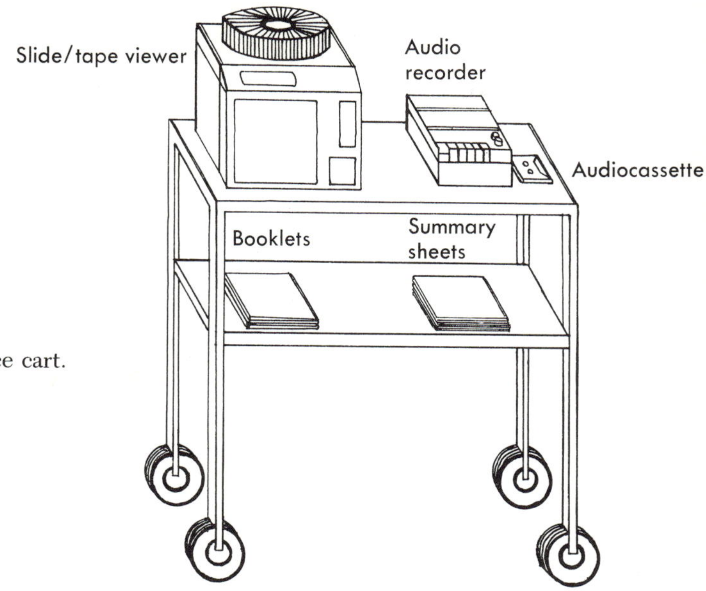

Fig. 3-8. Mobile in-service cart.

Self-contained units, as illustrated in Fig. 3-8, can be placed on mobile in-service carts, enabling the staff to use the instructional materials on their respective units at any time their priorities permit.

The amount of training time saved by a slide-tape program cannot be overstressed. This medium is probably one of the most cost-effective vehicles available to meet today's training needs. The following example illustrates this point:

> One of the responsibilities of the discharge planning department at a certain hospital is to provide recently hired nurses with an orientation to their role in the discharge planning program. Four times a year, three staff people from the discharge planning department present a six-hour session. Additional in-service sessions are held frequently throughout the year to educate other persons from multiple disciplines. After assessing the learning needs, establishing the program's learning objectives, and selecting teaching strategies, the discharge planning department decided to produce a slide-tape program. This program presented the philosophy and goals of the discharge planning program, described the multidisciplinary approach to communication, and identified the discharge planning consultants and their individual job responsibilities. After one year the department realized that it had saved approximately 200 hours of training time. Translated into dollars, this amount is sizable.

If media specialists are available at your institution, they can assist you with the development of a slide-tape program. Cost-effectiveness would increase if a few hospitals produced a program together and shared the equipment.

This chapter unfortunately does not have the space to discuss the actual creation of a slide-tape program; however, when developing the program script, keep in mind the following points:

- Avoid a lengthy narration
- Avoid the inclusion of too many concepts
- Reinforce or summarize thoroughly

- Encourage learner participation and involvement by asking questions relating to the learner's experiences or observations

Scripts may require two or three drafts before they are polished. Remember to keep the narrative conversational in style, and use vocabulary appropriate to the audience.

Visual materials carry the weight of the presentation and allow the narrative to flow along with the slides. Slides of individual providers carrying through the discharge planning process provide an important educational opportunity. For more information, readers are referred to Eastman Kodak's excellent how-to booklet *Planning and Producing Slide Programs*[8] and Jerald Kemp's *Planning and Producing Audiovisual Materials*.[14]

SUMMARY

In summation, the following guidelines will be helpful in the creation and implementation of a multidisciplinary discharge planning in-service education program:

1. Assess the learner's former *knowledge levels* before the in-service education program begins.
2. Develop measurable *behavioral objectives* to meet the stated goal(s).
3. Select the *teaching strategy* based on the established behavioral objectives.
4. Develop an *evaluation mechanism* to assess the cognitive and affective objectives of the overall program.
5. Choose personnel responsible for facilitating the discharge planning in-service program who have the expertise and knowledge to be *effective role models* for the discharge planning process.
6. Be flexible in all phases of the in-service education program. For example, if the staff members cannot attend the program, go to them via *mobile in-service carts*.
7. Actively involve participants in the *total learning experience*—cognitively, emotionally, and physically.

REFERENCES

1. Barbour, A., and Goldberg, A.: Interpersonal communication: teaching strategies and resources, New York, 1974, Speech Communication Association.
2. Bevis, E. O.: Curriculum building in nursing: a process, ed. 2, St. Louis, 1978, The C. V. Mosby Co.
3. Bloom, B. S., Handbook 1: Cognitive domain. In Bloom, B. S., editor: Taxonomy of educational objectives: the classification of educational goals, New York, 1956, David McKay Co.
4. Brown, J., Lewis, R., and Harderoad, F.: AV instruction: technology, media, and methods, ed. 4, New York, 1973, McGraw-Hill Book Co.
5. Bullough, R.: Creating instructional materials, ed. 2, Columbus, Ohio, 1978, Charles E. Merrill Publishing Co.
6. Davies, J.: Competency-based learning: technology, management and design, New York, 1973, McGraw-Hill Book Co.

7. Davis, J.: Teaching strategies for the college classroom, Boulder, Colo. 1976, Westview Press.
8. Eastman Kodak Motion Picture and Education Markets Division: Planning and producing slide programs, Rochester, N.Y., 1975, Eastman Kodak Co.
9. Gerlach, V., and Ely, D.: Teaching and media: a systematic approach, Englewood Cliffs, N.J., 1971, Prentice-Hall.
10. Gorham, R.: Systems approach to education: a model for the design of instructional materials. In Zalatimo, A., and Sleeman, P., editors: A systems approach to learning environments, Roselle, N.J., 1975, Meded Projects.
11. Instructional Development Institute, National Special Media Institute, Washington, D.C., 1975, Media Specialist Program, Division of Educational Technology, Bureau of Libraries and Educational Technology, Office of Education.
12. Isaac, S.: Handbook in research and evaluation, San Diego, 1971, Robert R. Knapp, Publisher.
13. Kemp, J.: Evaluating program outcomes, Audiovis. Instruc., vol. 23, no. 8, November, 1978.
14. Kemp, J.: Planning and producing audiovisual materials, New York, 1975, Thomas Y. Crowell Co.
15. Kibler, R., Barker, L., and Miles, D.: Behavioral objectives and instruction, Boston, 1970, Allyn & Bacon.
16. Kramer, M.: Reality shock: why nurses leave nursing, St. Louis, 1974, The C. V. Mosby Co.
17. Kratwohl, D., Bloom, B., and Masia, B.: Handbook 2: Affective domain. In Bloom, B. S., editor: Taxonomy of educational objectives: the classification of educational goals, New York, 1964, David McKay Co.
18. LeDuc, M. L., and Price, R. D.: Diabetes education program development, East Lansing, 1978, Department of Community Health Science, College of Human Medicine and Osteopathic Medicine, Michigan State University.
19. Osgood, C., Suci, G., and Tannenbaum, P.: The measurement of meaning, Urbana, Ill., 1957, University of Illinois Press.
20. Soulier, J.: Are you wasting time on your handouts? Audiov. Instruc. **24**(4):18-19, 1979.
21. Thiagarajan, S.: Relevance check for self-instructional packages, Audiov. Instruc. **20**(9), 1975.
22. Uustal, D., and Read, D.: A nursing challenge: searching for values, N. Scituate, Mass., Duxbury Press. In press.
23. Uustal, D.: Values and ethics: considerations in nursing practice, 1978. Privately published by author, 8 Moss Lane, Amherst, Mass. 01002.
24. Wollensak Manufacturing Co.: Developing cassette/slide presentations, St. Paul, Minn., 1978, Wollensak/3M Company. Privately published manual for workshop use.

ADDITIONAL READINGS

American Hospital Association: Media handbook, Atlanta, 1978, Bureau of Health Education, Department of Health, Education, and Welfare.

Bullough, R., and Duane, F.: Utilizing the tape recorder in teaching (slide/tape program), Salt Lake City, 1975, Media Systems.

Erickson, C., and Curl, D.: Fundamentals of teaching with audiovisual technology, New York, 1972, Macmillan Publishing Co.

Gagne, R.: Conditions of learning, ed. 2, New York, 1965, Holt, Rinehart and Winston.

Minor, E., and Frye, H.: Techniques for producing visual media, New York, 1970, McGraw-Hill Book Co.

Simon, S.: Meeting yourself halfway, Niles, Ill., 1974, Argus Communications.

Simon, S., Howe, L., and Kirschenbaum, H.: Values clarification: a handbook of teaching strategies, New York, 1972, Hart Publishing Co.

Smith, M.: A practical guide to values clarification, La Jolla, Calif., 1977, University Associates.

Wittich, W., and Schuller, C.: Instructional technology: its nature and use, ed. 6, New York, 1979, Harper & Row, Publishers.

CHAPTER 4

Establishment of an association of discharge planning consultants

SANDRA AUSTIN

Changing trends in health care have resulted in the training of health professionals dedicated to providing expertise in discharge planning. My involvement in this area during the past ten years has convinced me that similar problems are encountered by discharge planning consultants as they assume this new role. Most of these difficulties are based on situations in which role diffusion and role ambiguity exist among team members.

This chapter will identify some of the reasons that discharge planning consultants encounter role ambiguity and role conflict and will discuss how these problems lead to the natural evolvement of reference groups.

The establishment of reference groups is the first step toward organizing an association of discharge planners. As a member and officer of the Boston Regional Continuing Care Nurses' Association, I have shared in the initial development of this organization. I have used this experience to outline the benefits to be derived from formal organization and the methods that might be utilized in the structuring of an association of discharge planning consultants.

The process of developing a new role often results in ambiguity, lack of clear-cut role patterns, and role conflict among health team members. An organization of discharge planning consultants can help to reduce the negative effects of role negotiation and provide a reference group to solve problems and reinforce role assignments.

WHY A NEW ROLE?

The concept of continuity of care between the hospital and the community is not new. For years, nurses and social workers have worked as partners in an attempt to identify and plan for patients' continuing care needs. This partnership was generally based on clear-cut role definitions made possible by the simpler health care system of the past. During recent years, trends supporting the concepts of health promotion, prevention, and maintenance have led to the mushrooming of health care resources designed to increase the public's options in obtaining health services. As the system has become more complicated (through the development of regulations, reimbursement systems, and criteria for levels of care), the ability of the nurse and social worker to continue to effectively assume this role as part of their general job description has begun to decrease. The result is a need to designate a person or multidisciplinary team to become knowledgeable regarding the maze of community-based services and to coordinate primary provider efforts in the pursuit of continuity of care.

The basic goals of discharge planning consultants generally revolve around the need to increase hospital staff awareness of community health services and to assist hospital staff in identifying patients who require comprehensive aftercare planning. In some instances these goals will be consistent with an already existing multidisciplinary approach to discharge planning. In other instances the discharge planning consultant will be viewed as an intruder and usurper of the legitimate role of existing hospital professionals. A lack of guidelines regarding role responsibility often leads to a situation of role ambiguity between the social worker, continuing care consultant, staff nurse, and physician as each attempts to integrate his or her perceived role into the team concept. The attempt by each discipline to define its practice area is based on a mutual need to define responsibility and accountability within the discharge planning process. Through established role definitions, an orderly, interactive process can evolve that will maximize the expertise of each team member toward the goal of quality discharge planning.

DEVELOPMENT OF DISCHARGE PLANNING CONSULTANT ROLE

The role of the discharge planning consultant may be determined in several ways. First, a traditional job description may be developed by the administration within the employing institution. Second, the role may evolve as a result of the expectations of other health care givers. A third set of role qualifiers may come from reference groups such as state nursing or social work organizations, special interest groups, or community affiliations. A fourth set of influencing factors are the consultants' own perceptions of what constitutes appropriate role responsibilities. As one can easily see, consistency among role qualifiers leads to role stability, and a lack of consistency breeds role ambiguity or role conflict.[1]

Based on the above process of role allocation, many factors intervene to contribute to a system of undifferentiated roles among professionals. Discussion of some of those factors follows.

Nurses and social workers often enter positions in discharge planning with only a vague idea of what their role should be. Job descriptions related to this function are generally not available, and only a few institutions employ persons qualified to assist in its development. Research has not yet defined this scope of practice or measured discharge planning outcomes; thus consultants are responsible for developing their own degree of specialization without a familiar pattern or expertise to draw from.

In the absence of clear-cut role patterns, nurses and social workers utilize whatever cues are avilable to formulate job descriptions. Through trial and error and appraisal and reappraisal, individual philosophies of discharge planning are established. During the process of role negotiation, colleagues' expectations often conflict with the discharge planning consultant's perceived role. In some instances this role is viewed as a duplication of already established functional roles or as usurpation of power that rightfully belongs to another team member.

When such circumstances arise, it is important for the persons involved to identify the discrepancies that exist between colleagues' expectations of each other. Meetings can be called to clarify each member's role and responsibility, thus resolving the problem. In some cases it may be advisable to request that an outside party assist in clarifying the formal role assignment of each team member.

Resistance to change is frequently apparent in the relationship between the physician and the discharge planning consultant. Physicians, through education and training, are traditionally opposed to changes that delegate any additional authority to other team members. Nurses, social workers, and others providing judgments about the need for continuous health services are often criticized for attempting to monitor or influence physician practice.

Role conflict also results when the hospital nursing staff views the discharge planning consultant as assuming a function that has traditionally been theirs. To some nurses, sharing this discharge planning function means a loss of power and control in an area that is their rightful domain.

In such circumstances it may first be necessary to assist the nursing staff in understanding the concepts basic to a multidisciplinary approach to patient care. If information is provided and the staff members are supported during their transition from a more traditional to a multidisciplinary approach, much misunderstanding and displacement anxiety can be avoided.

Lack of clearly established role functions also leads to role ambiguity between nurse consultants and social work consultants. Coordination of the discharge planning process has been, in most instances, the responsibility of the social service department. When nurses have entered into this process their respective areas of responsibility have often been unclear to both the nurse and the social worker.

In some instances, meeting between social workers and nurse discharge planners to review the changing health care legislation will help to identify reasons that nurses have entered the discharge planning field. State and federal reimbursement systems are often based on a concept of levels of care, that is, skilled versus nonskilled services. Since the determination regarding what constitutes a skilled versus a nonskilled service is usually based on health care and nursing needs, involvement by nurses can assist the social worker in identifying what resources will be available to the client after discharge.

In an attempt to clarify roles, a series of meetings to discuss aspects of the discharge planning process can help to identify the areas of expertise that are shared by both disciplines, as well as those areas that are specific to each. In this way all members gain a better understanding of one another's concerns and expectations, which will support the process of role negotiation.

GROWTH OF REFERENCE GROUPS

Although the problems identified are common to any person entering a new role, not all discharge planning consultants will experience difficulties in all areas. In many instances the discharge planning consultant will be viewed as an effective health care resource person, and frequently the nurse and social work consultant will blend their expertise and provide mutual role support. Generally, however, both disciplines will experience a lack of peer support within their institution of employment. Finding few persons within their work setting capable of sharing the frustrations and rewards of the discharge planning consultant role, members of both disciplines begin to experience feelings of professional isolation. The result is that both social workers and nurses actively search outside the institution for a reference group capable of meeting or supporting their professional needs.

In their search for a reference group, nurses involved in discharge planning often turned to the special-interest groups of their state nursing association. In this setting many common areas of concern were shared and information was gained, but the goals of these groups did not always address the specific professional activities and problems that were of primary interest to nurses employed as discharge planning consultants.

Through cooperative health efforts between hospitals, the number of nurse discharge planning contacts begin to increase. From these contacts an informal communication network may develop for the purpose of sharing resource information. In this manner, nurses slowly begin to identify with a peer group involved in similar operational and professional difficulties.

During 1975 a small group of Boston-area nurse discharge planning consultants initiated informal group meetings for the purpose of collection and dissemination of information. These meetings led to the establishment of common goals, one of which was a group effort to develop role clarity by specifically defining the role of a nurse discharge planning consultant. Through the process of assessment and reassessment of tasks, consultants became resources for one another, and the group became a resource for new consultants entering the field. As these nurses gained experience, role ambiguities and conflicts began to resolve, thus freeing energy to be used in other areas. This energy was directed toward problems resulting from the expansion of the health care delivery system. Although consultants new to the field still needed to focus on identity issues, an increasing number of members began to look toward the group to meet goals that could not be met through individual efforts. It was believed that collective action was the mechanism by which changes in health care could be effected on a statewide basis.

Although there are many ways to structure any formal organization, I have drawn on my experience with the Boston Regional nurse coordinators group to identify one structure that meets the purpose and goals of an association of discharge planning consultants.

The following discussion first identifies the rationale for development of an association and then describes a method that may be used to define its formal structure. Each component of the structure is then further defined by presenting its rationale and specific ways in which it may be developed.

METHODS OF ORGANIZING AN ASSOCIATION

Formal organization of discharge planning consultants provides a mechanism whereby interests and energies of a collective whole may be directed toward the attainment of individual and group goals.

A committee to develop proposed bylaws should be nominated and elected by the membership-at-large. The functions of this committee are to (1) determine the basic rules relating to the principles of organization, (2) prescribe how the organization should function, and (3) develop the rules the organization considers so important that they cannot be changed without the majority vote by a specified number of persons.

Once the bylaws are developed, they should be presented to the membership one meeting in advance of when they are to be submitted to a vote. This allows members time to consider each article and to make arrangements to be present at the time of bylaw enactment. At this meeting the bylaws should be reviewed, article by article, and approved only after gaining a two-thirds affirmative vote of the membership.

During bylaw development the general nature of the subjects to be addressed include but are not limited to (1) name of the organization, (2) organization objectives, (3) membership definition, (4) types and responsibilities of officers, (5) meeting frequency, (6) types of committees, and (7) process for making amendments.

The bylaws should define the *purpose* and *functions* of the organization in terms that reflect member goals. Since discharge planning consultants tend to be somewhat heterogeneous in background, education, and job responsibility, the organization should define its purpose and functions in terms broad enough to encompass a variety of goals.

An example of this type of definition is found in the stated purpose of the Boston Regional group: "To enhance the quality of health care services for patients with continuing care needs by: (1) sharing information regarding current health policies; (2) acting as an organized vehicle for change in the health care system as they effect continuing care services; (3) sharing resources and knowledge; (4) serving as a resource for new discharge planning consultants; (5) providing liaisons to other health-related groups."[2]

Membership

Method of development

Constituency. The bylaws should identify qualifications or eligibility for membership within the association. Areas to be considered when determining eligibility include the size of the group, the region to be represented, and the mix of health professionals to be included. Some organizations have chosen to limit their membership to those persons working in acute care settings, and others have limited membership to just one discipline, such as nursing or social services.

My view is that the most effective organization is one that utilizes and integrates the expertise of both social workers and nurse discharge planning consultants in pursuit of improved continuity of care. I maintain that there are greater benefits to be derived by the collective whole when an organization utilizes a partnership approach.

Type of membership. Once membership constituency has been determined, a decision must be made regarding the type of membership preferred. The institutional membership entitles consultants from the same institution to attend meetings and participate on task force and special interest groups, but it limits the voting rights to one collective vote. An individual membership allows each consultant the same privileges regardless of institutional affiliation.

Frequently during the developmental stage of group organization there is concern that a few hospitals that employ several discharge planning consultants will unduly influence the decision-making process of the group. So that decisions will reflect each discharge planning system, an institutional membership is often adopted.

In the three years of my experience, the Boston Regional group found that this concern never became a reality.

Officers

Rationale for types of officers. The bylaws should specify the offices required to carry out group functions and the method by which officers shall be appointed or elected. For example, the Boston Regional Continuing Care Nurses' Association has identified a need for four officers: chairperson, vice-chairperson, secretary, and treasurer.

Method of development. A nominating committee should be formed for the purpose of nominating candidates for each office. Elections by ballot with announcement of results should take place at the annual meeting, designated as such, for the purpose of electing officers and collecting annual reports from task force members.

The duties of the officers should be described by the bylaws so that problems in interpretation of the rights or responsibilities of office are reduced. The following discussion suggests duties of officers.

Chairperson. The chairperson has the following responsibilities:

1. Presides at all meetings of the consultants.

   This duty involves the preparation and dissemination of meeting agendas far enough in advance for members to determine or research specific areas of interest. It also includes advance distribution of material which will be used in discussion or on which voting will take place.

   It is the chairperson's responsibility to structure the meetings to include issues or concerns shared by the majority of members. Since many of these issues are not resolved during any one meeting, it is helpful for the chairperson to briefly summarize past discussions and decisions, as well as to assist members in continuing to move toward resolution of an issue.

   During the process of issue resolution, it may be necessary to refocus communication toward the problem to be resolved, redirect the focus when conversations have reached an impasse, summarize the issue when it has been adequately discussed, and reiterate the decisions and commitments for action.

   It is also the role of the chairperson and other officers to provide and maintain an environment conducive to group interaction. It may at times be necessary to control overactive members or to support and draw out those less able to state their position.
2. Appoints standing and special committees with the approval of the other officers.
3. Fills vacancies, by appointment, in the standing and special committees if less than two thirds of term has been completed.
4. Acts as an ex-officio member of all committees except the committee on nominations.

Vice-chairperson. The vice-chairperson has the following responsibilities:

1. Performs the duties of the chairperson in that person's absence.
2. Becomes the chairperson in case of a vacancy in that office.
3. Functions as an ex-officio member of committees as appointed by the chairperson.

My perception of the typically designated responsibilities of this office is that there is a tendency, by role definition, to underutilize the leadership ability of this officer. Functions appropriate to the vice-chairperson's role are those of gathering background data and supporting information on agenda topics, assisting in structuring the work to be accomplished, supporting members in developing an effective interaction process, and assisting in directing group behavior.

Inherent in the responsibility of any office is the need to be responsive to the problems and concerns of constitutents. Each officer has a duty to maintain an ongoing evaluation of the effectiveness of the group process, and to initiate actions designed to promote improved responses.

Secretary. Since one purpose of the consultant's group is to provide current information to its members, it is imperative that an effective information network be established. This may be accomplished through the office of the secretary, who has the following duties:

1. Obtains an accurate list of the names, addresses, and telephone numbers of the members
2. Notifies members of the time and place of all meetings
3. Keeps minutes of all meetings or, when absent, makes arrangements for a replacement
4. Conducts general correspondence
5. Preserves all papers, letters, and transactions
6. Furnishes committees with all papers referred to them
7. Keeps a current file of annual reports from committees

Treasurer. The duties of the treasurer are as follows:

1. Takes charge of all money, such as money in a bank designated by the membership
2. Pays out money designated by the membership
3. Reports to the membership the financial standing when requested and makes a full report at the annual meeting
4. Applies for IRS tax-exempt status

Dues

The bylaws should specify the required fees and dues, the date when payable, the date when dues are considered in arrears, and the penalty of dues in arrears.

Rationale for dues. Membership and voting privileges should be dependent on the payment of dues. This ensures that adequate financial resources will be available for debts incurred and for program planning.

Method of development. As in most nonprofit organizations, annual dues should be determined according to anticipated operating expenses. These fees should ensure revenue sufficient to cover postage and the mailing of minutes and bulletins, membership dues of agencies in which the organization desires membership, the cost of obtaining desired resource publication, honorariums for speakers, and money for initiating educational conferences.

Meetings

The bylaws should specify the type, frequency, and length of association meetings.

Rationale for meetings. The assembly of members is necessary to transact business, share information regarding health care policy, and make decisions enabling the organization to act as a vehicle for change.

Method of development. The basic components (agenda) of these meetings should include the reading and approval of minutes, reports of officers and standing committees, liaison reports, task force reports, and unfinished and new business.

A specific meeting location may be established, or a practice of rotating meeting locations may be adopted. Rotating meetings among member hospitals is advantageous for two reasons. First, it provides consultants with the opportunity to share current information about their institutions. Second, since membership may include persons from a wide geographic area, rotating locations ensures that certain members are not consistently asked to travel long distances to participate in meetings.

In addition to regularly scheduled monthly meetings, the bylaws should include provision for the calling of special meetings to allow the membership to deal with important matters that arise between regularly scheduled meetings.

The bylaws should identify one regular business meeting to be known as the annual meeting. This annual meeting should be designated for the election of officers and the collection of final committee reports. A review of the past year's events allows the membership to refocus on group goals and reestablish priorities for the coming year.

Affiliations

The continuing care organization should develop affiliations with other health-related associations.

Rationale for affiliations. It is advantageous to form close affiliations with other associations involved in the health delivery system so that members are able to remain knowledgeable regarding changes in health care practices. Many of these health care resources provide up-to-date information that helps discharge planning consultants to maintain awareness of current health care trends.

Method of development. A committee or task force should be developed to explore the possibility of various affiliation relationships. Once information has been gathered, the membership can evaluate potential benefits to be derived from association membership. The following is an example of three associations with which the Boston Regional group has elected to form formal affiliations.

Affiliations

State hospital association. One of the most valuable affiliations of the Boston Regional continuing care group is with the Massachusetts Hospital Association. Membership ensures access to an array of weekly and monthly publications relating to state, federal, and community actions that impact on the hospital system. The following are some of the more informative publications:

1. Issue papers, which depict major changes in the hospital role within the health care industry and from which one can anticipate future trends that will influence the health care delivery system
2. Bulletins, which provide up-to-date information regarding changes in state and federal reimbursement systems
3. Legal and legislative reports, which provide a series of summaries depicting the status of legislative proposals that impact on health care resources
4. Reprints of health care publications, such as the report of the National Health Planning Committee

5. *Monday Reports,* which are weekly newsletters that update the activities of the Massachusetts Hospital Association

In addition to ensuring the availability of numerous publications, the Massachusetts Hospital Association gives its affiliates access to professional advisers who are able to supply information on areas of interest, such as court decisions.

State public health association. Another organizational membership that has proved useful is the state public health association.

This organization consists of persons whose purpose is to "improve health conditions, promote health care as a human right, and secure optimal community, personal, and environmental health."[3]

Membership is open to persons or institutions whose primary interest lies within the public health field. The association is thus a meeting ground for professionals involved in both the health care delivery and health care administration fields.

The Massachusetts State Public Health Association is divided into sections, each section being responsible for developing position papers on issues related to its area. Each section is also responsible for developing informational and educational programs of current interest to public health members.

Benefits derived from a state public health association membership may include access to information via the current monthly newsletter, availability of ongoing educational programs, and the opportunity to share discharge planning concerns in a multidisciplinary forum.

Professional associations. Although there is not enough space in this chapter to outline all the benefits that professional organizations provide for its members, there are several services that specifically support the growth and development of a new nursing or social worker role. These services increase and validate the body of knowledge that is unique to its constituents. They may also provide education to its practitioners and set standards of practice based on ethical principles. Since the professional association can become the legislative spokesman for an entire discipline, the professional association can impact on policy decisions affecting the political, legal, and economic sphere of the profession. An additional benefit includes access to a medium of information exchange on both a formal and an informal basis.

Liaison officers

Consultants should be appointed or elected to maintain liaisons between the discharge planning organization and other health related groups.

Rationale for liaison officers. The present health care delivery system encompasses a wide variety of organizations and practitioners dedicated to providing quality health care. Discharge planning consultants, as part of this evolving and dynamic system, share goals and objectives that are similar to those of other agencies. At an organizational level it is possible, through a liaison system, to identify similar objectives and work cooperatively on issues of mutual concern.

Method of development. It is often beneficial to develop liaisons with certain agencies such as the local home health agency, the welfare department, or a specific department within the state department of public health. Liaison officers can facilitate communication whereby each organization is kept apprised of current changes related to the other's field. They may also initiate joint problem-solving activities, as well as assist in coordinating common endeavors. A liaison officer maintains communication with other groups in the following ways:

1. Identifies a contact person within the related health care agency
2. An introductory meeting scheduled during the first month of the association's calendar year, performs the following functions:
   a. Explains the purpose of the discharge planning consultant's association
   b. Provides the agency with a copy of the association's membership and an outline of standing committees
   c. Defines the association's goals and objectives for that year
   d. Obtains information from the agency that would be useful to the discharge planning consultants' association
3. Maintains continued contact, on a quarterly basis, via telephone or meetings with the agency, and calls meetings as necessary
4. Writes reports of liaison activities for the chairperson or membership-at-large after each of the quarterly contacts
5. Provides recommendations from the discharge planning consultants' association to the agency as necessary, and relays feedback from the agency regarding these recommendations
6. Presents a summarized written and verbal report at the annual meeting[2]

Liaison contacts that have proved helpful to the Boston Regional consultants' group are the Massachusetts Department of Elder Affairs, Massachusetts Public Health Council, Massachusetts Federation of of Nursing Homes, Council of Elders, Department of Public Welfare, Blue Cross/Blue Shield, Department of Public Health, Social Work Directors Association, and the Massachusetts State Nursing Association.

Standing committees

The bylaws should specify (1) the types of committees deemed necessary to function in behalf of the association, (2) the method by which committee membership shall be determined, and (3) the scope and limitations of committee authority.

Rationale for standing committees. A standing committee is able to focus on a particular continuing concern of the association. In addition, a small number of persons are able to give a task more detailed attention than the larger group can manage.

Method of development. The alternatives available for committee selection include appointment by the chairperson, election by ballot, or nomination from the floor. The Boston Regional group identified the chairperson as being responsible for choosing committee membership. My experience has shown me that consultants will volunteer to work in areas where they have vested interests or in which they have applicable knowledge and experience. Since the voluntary commitment of time and energy usually precludes the participation of all members except those who are dedicated to accomplishing committee goals, this system of committee appointment is recommended.

The standing committees that I view as an asset to a discharge planning association include a legislative and lobbying committee, a continuing education committee, and a resource committee. A brief description of each follows.

Legislative and lobbying committee

Rationale for legislative and lobbying committee. The purpose of this committee is to review and respond to legislation that impacts on discharge planning.

Method of development. The legislative and lobbying committee should have a chairperson to coordinate the activity of its members, a work force to review legislation proposals, and liaison (e.g., area health planning meetings).

Several organizations (state hospital association, nursing and health council, etc.) employ full-time legislative staff to review and make recommendations regarding proposed health legislation. The discharge planning legislative and lobbying committee often relies on another group's screening process to pass along information on current health legislation. With the preliminary screening done, the members can direct their attention to issues that impact on discharge planning.

Once legislative reviews have occurred, the committee should present brief informative programs to the membership regarding the potential effects of the health care legislation being considered. After gaining approval from the membership, this committee should develop formal position statements and provide oral testimony on current health care issues. The Boston Regional legislative and lobbying committee, as part of its work, has thus far accomplished the following:

1. Submitted written testimony at public hearings on draft proposals of an area health systems plan
2. Given testimony at the public hearing concerning home health agency services
3. Attended a meeting of the board of directors of a health planning council
4. Presented educational programs to the Boston Regional membership regarding proposed national health insurance legislation

Continuing education committee

Rationale for continuing education committee. The purpose of a continuing education committee is to develop educational programs designed to increase the growth and expertise of discharge planning consultants. Although there is an abundance of ongoing education programs, few have been created that are geared toward increasing the discharge planner's satisfaction, skills, and knowledge.

Method of development. The committee should consist of persons who have an interest in researching education needs and in developing new programs where none previously existed. The scope of education services may include the development of workshops, the coordination of education programs with other discharge planning consultant groups, and the development and maintenance of ongoing educational materials.

One of the most successful services of the Boston Regional group was the development of annual multidiscipline/multitopic educational programs geared toward interests identified by the membership. Following is a recipe for the development of such a program.

AGENDA. One method of developing program content is to request topic suggestions from the membership-at-large. The development of a program around those topics receiving the most requests will ensure the greatest number of conference participants.

SPEAKERS. Making decisions regarding choice of speakers and content to be included in topic presentation is a legitimate committee function. Under some circumstances the committee may choose experts from within the discharge planning consultants association. At other times it might be advantageous to choose outside speakers, but be sure to assess the association's internal membership resources first.

LOCATION. Before a conference meeting site is chosen, the following questions should be answered: How many participants does the conference intend to attract? From what geographic area will the majority of the participants come? What is the committee's work capacity in terms of time and commitment? Answers to these questions will determine the size, structure, and geographic location of the meeting site. Before the final choice is made, it is wise to explore several alternatives, since charges and services vary from place to place. Often hotels and motels provide complimentary meeting rooms, coffee, public address systems, blackboards, podiums, screens, and so forth in return for a designated number of luncheon commitments.

ADVERTISEMENT. The design and printing of the program are dependent on resources available to the committee. The utilization of the artistic talents of its members and gratuitous printing from hospital resources can provide an economical solution to financial constraints. In the event that a more sophisticated advertisement technique is required, the committee may elect to purchase the services of a local printing company.

COSTS. The cost of planning and implementing an education program is dependent on the individual characteristics of that program. Standard fees, regardless of the number of conference participants, usually include honorariums and payments for rental equipment, printing, and stamps. Costs that are dependent on participant attendance include fees for luncheons, meeting rooms, and parking facilities. During the planning stage the committee should make a careful assessment of anticipated costs and set the registration fee so that the revenue collected will be equal to the debt incurred.

EVALUATION. Since continuing education programs are designed to meet specific objectives, an evaluation tool should be developed to measure the success of that attempt. The committee members must therefore have a clear concept of program objectives. This concept should be shared with program speakers so that individual presentations contribute to the overall goals.

After completion of the program, each conference participant should be able to identify areas where learning has occurred as a result of conference participation. An evaluation tool should thus be developed to provide feedback about both the individual speaker and the effectiveness of the program as a whole.

Resource committee

Rationale for resource committee. Since discharge planning is a relatively new area of concentration, little written information is available to assist discharge planning consultants in structuring their programs or departments. A resource committee can gather data from existing discharge planning programs related to their structure and process of operation. This information can then be compiled into a resource manual to be utilized by discharge planning consultants in developing or evaluating their own discharge planning system.

Method of development. The responsibility of a resource committee is to gather information related to the structure and process of discharge planning departments within the identified geographic area. Information related to structure may include such items as size and type of institution, ratio of discharge planning consultants to hospital census, and place of discharge planning within the hospital's organization chart. Information related to process includes identification of job responsibilities; provision of either direct or consultation services; participation in multidisciplinary team conferences; obtaining of home care services, transportation, and long-term care placements; provision of discharge follow-up; and presentation of in-service education programs on discharge planning within an institution.

Access to this type of information allows members to review the functions of other discharge planning departments and to compare and contrast program goals. The ability to selectively compare programs that have similar operational difficulties may lend credibility to a consultant's attempts to initiate change.

Another function of the resource committee is to obtain information regarding individual discharge planning department protocols, assessment or evaluation tools, and documentation and statistical reporting mechanisms.

Task force committees

Rationale for task force committees. Task force committees usually develop in response to problems or situations identified by the membership as needing change. The assignment of a small group of persons to investigate a problem allows for maximum efficiency and economy, which are not possible in the larger-group setting.

Method of development. Design of the committee is usually dictated by the nature of the problem. Under some circumstances the membership will comprise persons within the association. In other circumstances the definition of the problem and actions necessary to bring about a resolution will dictate that other groups or disciplines be involved.

Total group concensus on any given issue is rare, and activities leading to change will most certainly be met by resistance from some groups. The task force can help to minimize this resistance by developing an open system of input, output, and feedback to the larger membership. The necessity of obtaining input is twofold: first, it serves to increase the data base available to the task force, and second, it serves as a means of building group acceptance for committee recommendations (few members will provide resistance to changes that are the result of their contribution). Since the efforts of the task force generally result in recommendations requiring change, it is imperative that this committee receive the official status and sanction of the membership. Output from the task force should consist of periodic oral or written progress reports.

CONCLUSION

Since discharge planning is a new area of concentration, consultants in discharge planning are faced with the task of building a base of knowledge and skills specific to this field. During the process of role development, ambiguity and role diffusion are often encountered. An organized association of discharge planning consultants can act as a reference group, provide support, and assist in the process of role clarification.

It is well recognized that a collective group is often more than the sum of its individual parts; thus an organized association of discharge planning consultants can accomplish more than can individuals working separately. By sharing information and defining problems from varying points of view, consultants gain a more complete perspective of health care issues. Collective action can then be initiated toward making needed changes within the health care system.

The ability of the association to function in an orderly, productive manner will be dependent on the development of a defined organizational structure and process. This may best be accomplished through the adoption of formal bylaws that define such areas as purpose and function, membership eligibility, establishment of affiliations, choice of officers, and formation of standing committees and task force committees necessary to accomplish group goals.

The development of an organized association of discharge planning consultants will ensure an orderly, interactive process whereby individual member interests contribute to collective group goals.

REFERENCES

1. Benne, K., and Bennis, W.: The role of the professional nurse, Am. J. Nurs. vol. 59, Feb., 1959.
2. Boston Regional Continuing Care Nurses' Association: Bylaws, 1978.
3. Massachusetts Public Health Association: Your Massachusetts Public Health Association, Boston, n.d., the Association.

ADDITIONAL READINGS

Bailey, J. T., and Claus, K. E.: Decision making in nursing: tools for change, St. Louis, 1975, The C. V. Mosby Co.

Miller, M. H., and Flynn, B. C., editors: Current perspectives in nursing: social issues and trends, vol. I, St. Louis, 1977, The C. V. Mosby Co.

Roberts, H. M.: Roberts' rules of order, Glenview, Ill., 1970, Scott, Foresman and Co.

Stevens, B. J.: The nurse as executive, Wakefield, Mass., 1975, Contemporary Publishers.

SECTION TWO

Management practices in discharge planning

"If I ordered a general to fly from one flower to another like a butterfly, . . . and if the general did not carry out the order that he had received, which one of us would be in the wrong?" the king demanded. "The general, or myself ?"

"You," said the little prince firmly.

"Exactly. One must require from each one the duty which each one can perform," the king went on. "Accepted authority rests first of all on reason."

The Little Prince
Antoine de Saint-Exupéry

Health care providers have continued to develop professional skills, but they have not integrated the principles of management into their practice. This becomes clear when current patterns of health care delivery in the United States are analyzed and one of the most pressing problems identified is the utilization of ineffec-

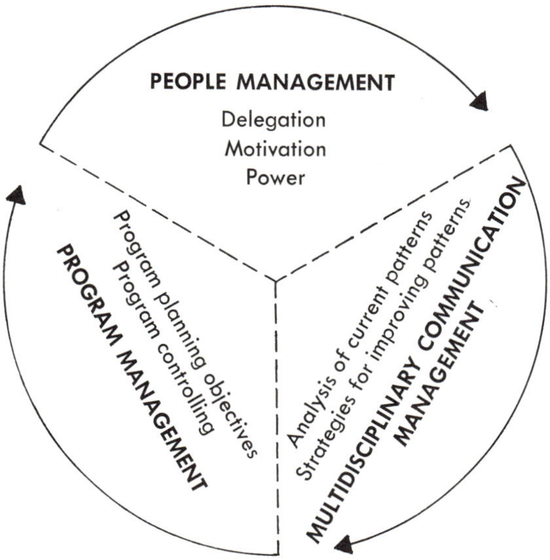

Model for management practices in discharge planning programs/departments.

tive management techniques.[1] Effective management is particularly important in discharge planning programs because of the many variables inherent in the discharge planning process.

A model proposed for management practices in discharge planning programs is shown in the illustration. Management is defined, in this context, as the process through which the objectives of the discharge planning program are accomplished by *human resources* utilizing the principal mechanism of *multidisciplinary communications*. The model has three components: program management, people management, and the management of multidisciplinary communications. Detailed discussion of each of these components is presented in the following three chapters.

REFERENCE

1. Longest, B. B.: Management practices for the health professional, Reston, Va., 1976, Reston Publishing Co., pp. 1-2.

CHAPTER 5

Program management in discharge planning

JANET PAPILE O'DAY
KATHLEEN M. McKEEHAN
CYNTHIA MacDONALD WALSH

The first component of the management model for discharge planning is program management. *Program management is the process which an organization or a department uses to accomplish its objectives.* The establishment of a discharge planning program has usually been based on an institution's need to improve or refine the continuity of patient care. This need generally arises from two sources: internally from perceived needs directly expressed by patients, families, or primary providers: and externally from specific regulatory agencies, community resources, or third-party payers. Regardless of the origin of the need, our experience has shown us that coordinated discharge planning leads to better continuity of care. For this reason, program management is essential in dealing with the multiple variables present in the discharge planning process.

One of the most important steps in program management is asking appropriate questions regarding the discharge planning process within an institution. Gertrude Stein once said, "Asking the right question is often more important than securing the right answers." Examples of management questions for a discharge planning program are as follows:

- What is a discharge planning program trying to accomplish?
- How will it go about accomplishing this goal?
- Who is responsible for planning discharge with patients?
- Who is responsible for coordinating discharge with patients?
- What procedures cover the discharge planning process?
- What community resources are available to patients after discharge?
- What is the rapport between your institution and community resources?
- Is discharge planning done with every patient (and documented)?
- What local and national regulations govern discharge planning for your institution?

All major regulatory bodies (such as the departments of public health and public welfare) that govern health care delivery systems address discharge planning within their regulations. Either fortunately or unfortunately (depending on one's point of view), most regulations appear to deal with the discharge planning process philosophically rather than concretely. There are, however, *some* concrete statements made about discharge planning. (Appendix B discusses federal and local legislation affecting discharge planning.)

In this chapter, two major aspects of program management will be discussed: *program planning* and *program controlling*. Encompassed within these sections are ten guidelines that are basic to the development and directing of discharge planning programs.

PROGRAM PLANNING

Program planning is deciding in advance *what* is to be done and *how* the institution will go about doing it.

1. *A formal planning committee should be established and should have the responsibility of designing the discharge planning program.*

Key administrative people from multidisciplinary departments should be represented on the planning committee. Commitments to a program are often cemented if individuals are allowed to take part in the building process. Examples of various departments from which there should be representation include nursing, social service, medicine, physical therapy, dietetics, occupational therapy, speech-language pathology, and hospital administration. The committee members should clearly understand the responsibility they have in designing the discharge planning program. Time limitations should be set up for the completion of the planning period, and the committee should meet consistently until the framework for the program has been completed.

2. *Environmental scanning should take place.*

An environmental scan identifies the primary elements within the institution and the community that impact on discharge planning. These elements are often problems that evolve from internal and external pressures. As an example of an internal pressure, the primary providers might state that they are unable to adequately plan discharge with patients because of their lack of knowledge regarding available community resources. As an example of an external pressure, Medicare administrators may have cited the hospital for poor documentation of discharge planning. An analysis of pressures related to discharge planning will help a discharge planning program set priorities when goals and objectives are established.

3. *There should be a strong commitment from hospital administration to create a discharge planning program.*

The best way to secure this commitment is to actively involve administrators in the planning committee. Open and honest communication among all departments is essential to the successful development of a discharge planning program.

4. *The program should be defined, and specific goals and objectives should be determined.*

Discharge planning is a relatively broad term; therefore it is important that the program be defined as concisely as possible. An example of a program definition might be as follows: *The discharge planning program is a hospital-based program that facilitates assessment, planning, and follow-up procedures by providing a multidisciplinary team approach to patients with post discharge needs*. The discharge planning program might be responsible for certain activities, such as making referrals to home health agencies and administering facility placement. The point being emphasized here is that parameters of the program should be defined so that the program's effectiveness can later be measured more readily.

Goals for the discharge planning program should be stated, and they should interface with the philosophy of the institution. For simplicity, a goal is defined as a statement identifying a perceived mission for which the program was created. An example of a goal could be the *integration of discharge planning as a priority within each primary provider's delivery of health care*.

Peter Drucker, a noted authority in management, coined the phrase "management by objectives" to illustrate the tremendous importance of setting objectives. An objective is a measurable action taken to achieve a goal. An example of an objective for the previously stated goal could be *to increase the comprehension of primary providers regarding discharge planning by functioning actively in multidisciplinary education programs*.

5. *A discharge planning program should be built on a multidisciplinary team concept.*

According to Rubin and associates, [3] noted authors in the management of health care teams, delivery of health care—as opposed to just the delivery of medical care, nursing care, or social care—*always* involves a team of persons from multiple disciplines. Representatives of the various disciplines should be *equal* in their position of planning discharge with patients; however, one specific discipline should be designated by the team to coordinate the discharge plan. The reader is encouraged to refer to Chapter 7, Management of Multidisciplinary Communication in Discharge Planning.

6. *Specific procedures should be developed to enhance a systematic approach to discharge planning.*

Procedures should be developed for each component of the discharge planning process: assessment, diagnosis, prescription, implementation, and evaluation. An example of a procedure for the combined *assessment* and *diagnosis* components is the case finding the staff accomplishes by screening patients during patient care rounds. Rounds on the units, conducted with primary providers and discharge planning consultants, provide an excellent opportunity to identify the discharge needs of patients. An example of the procedure used in the *prescription* component is the review of available community resources found in a manual kept on each patient-care unit. An example of a procedure in the *implementation* component is an outline of the specific role of persons from multiple disciplines in processing a referral to a home health agency. An example of a procedure in the *evaluation* component is the inclusion of a follow-up letter with the referral to a community agency. Certain procedures, such as those involving documentation, apply to all components of the discharge planning process. As an example, the discharge problems and plans for each patient might be listed on the medical record and on the nursing Kardex. Procedures covering the documentation of discharge plans often have two effects: (1) they hold primary providers accountable to the patient for discharge planning and (2) they provide concrete data for program audits.

PROGRAM CONTROLLING

Longest once wrote, "If the plans that are made to meet organizational objectives were always conceived and executed flawlessly by a perfectly structured organization where perfect coordination was achieved under the direction of an omnipotent leader, there would be no need for control."[2] Sadly, we do not exist in Nirvana; therefore control systems are needed to ensure that plans are being met. This section of the chapter will offer guidelines for controlling discharge planning programs.

7. *An advisory committee should be established and should include representation from the institution, community resources, and consumers.*

Advisory committees often evolve as an extension of planning committees. As the planning phase of a discharge planning program comes to a close, certain members from multiple disciplines should remain to advise in the ongoing development of the program. An advisory committee can provide three linkages: (1) a linkage to ensure that a multidisciplinary approach exists, as stated in the planning guidelines, (2) a linkage to community agencies to ensure open lines of communication, and (3) a linkage to consumers to ensure a feedback mechanism in delivery of care.

8. *Management data should be collected on a consistent basis to provide a profile of the discharge planning program as it develops.*

The most fundamental tool for control is data collection. The information collected and the system utilized to gather this information may differ from institution to institution, depending in part on staffing limitation and access to data processing. Examples of two data collection forms are located in Figs. 5-1 and 5-2.

A straightforward measurement of statistical data is presented in Fig. 5-1. It can be utilized to analyze a change in the number of referrals to long-term care

	Referrals	Oct	Nov	Dec	Jan	Feb	Mar	Apr	May	Jun	Jul	Aug	Sep	Total
Home health agencies	Boston VNA													
	Brookline VNA													
	Other VNA													
Facility placements	Skilled													
	Intermediate													
	Rest home													
Day care centers	Day care centers, adult													
	Day care centers, infant													
	Total													
														Grand total

Fig. 5-1. Frequency and distribution of patient referrals.

Reason for referral	Age	Sex	Medical diagnosis	Referral agency	Level of care	Source of payment	Living situation
Patient discharge problem, e.g., nursing diagnosis, social service diagnosis, and other multidisciplinary diagnoses							

Fig. 5-2. Profile of patients referred to home health agencies.

(LTC) facilities and community agencies. Such a change may indicate, perhaps, that (1) there is an increased work load on the discharge planning staff and that the need for additional personnel should be evaluated; (2) there are busy seasons for the department, which would affect vacation schedules; (3) there are trends in the use of community resources that should be considered in state and local health planning; and (4) there is an increased availability of services in the community.

A more sensitive table is shown in Fig. 5-2, which provides a way by which trends of change may be viewed over time. A place to list the discharge problems of patients is provided in Fig. 5-2. The data might be difficult to obtain unless an institution has adopted a taxonomy for patient discharge problems. One institution adopted the national list of nursing diagnoses for referrals to nursing agencies, and it further computerized and studied patient discharge problems over a period of time.[1] If an institution knew the most prevalent discharge problems of its patients, it could identify the need for specific community services.

It is to the advantage of discharge planning consultants to develop statistical systems that will serve the purpose of the program and provide the basic data required by the regulatory agencies. These agencies often request data that define the patient population in terms of such factors as age, insurance coverage, level of care, and utilization of community resources.

9. *Follow-up should be built into the program for purposes of evaluating the plan of care.*

Follow-up fulfills two functions: (1) it provides a mechanism for evaluating plans of care and (2) it provides support to employees of community agencies who may feel isolated from a team approach as they deliver their care. When large numbers of referrals to community resources (e.g., home health agencies and nursing homes) are involved, one of the best mechanisms for follow-up is a level of care system developed jointly by persons from various disciplines. A level of care system categorizes patients according to intensive, intermediate, and minimum levels of care need. Postdischarge conferences with community agencies are then set up to discuss patients with the greatest need.

Another strategy for follow-up could be the inclusion of a follow-up sheet in the referral. The program could request that the community agency mail back a written follow-up note that could be shared with primary providers. Some form of follow-up should be instituted in all discharge planning programs. If the numbers of referrals appear to be too large for an individual follow-up on all referrals, at least a statistically significant number of referrals, randomly selected, should be chosen for follow-up.

10. *An evaluation of the discharge planning program should be made at least once a year.*

Program evaluation in discharge planning is definitely in its embryo stages. Since there are so many variables affecting the discharge planning process, it is difficult to isolate each variable and to measure the program as a whole. There is, however, at least one valid approach to evaluating a discharge planning program: the measurement of objectives.

For example, one objective of the discharge planning program might be that a discharge plan be documented on each patient's medical record. An audit could then be conducted to identify whether this objective is being met. When an audit is performed, medical records are pulled at random and predetermined questions are answered by the auditor. The questions might include the following: How many days elapsed between the date of admission and the first mention of discharge planning? Were the discharge *problems* clearly documented? Was the discharge *plan* clearly documented? Did the plan address all the discharge problems identified? The results of such an audit will provide the institution with the information needed to evaluate how well the program is meeting its objective.

SUMMARY

In summation, program management encompasses ten guidelines. These guidelines provide a format for the analysis of relevant present, past, and probable future information that enables an institution to establish viable objectives for planning and controlling a discharge planning program.

REFERENCES

1. Gordon, M., Sweeney, M. A., and McKeehan, K. M.: Nursing diagnosis: looking at its use in the clinical area, Am. J. Nurs. **80**:672-674, April, 1980.
2. Longest, B. B.: Management practices for the health professional, Reston, Va., 1976, Reston Publishing Co.
3. Rubin, I., Plovnick, M., and Fry, R.: Improving the corrdination of care: a program for health team development, Cambridge, Mass., 1975, Ballinger Publishing Co.

ADDITIONAL READINGS

Donovan, H. M.: Nursing service administration: managing the enterprise, St. Louis, 1975, The C. V. Mosby Co.

Stevens, W. F.: Management and leadership in nursing, New York, 1978, McGraw-Hill Book Co.

CHAPTER 6

People management in discharge planning

CYNTHIA MacDONALD WALSH
JANET PAPILE O'DAY
KATHLEEN M. McKEEHAN

The second component of the model of management practices in discharge planning is people management. For purposes of this chapter, "people management" will be defined as *the art of drawing out the individual strengths of others and functionalizing them in such a way as to accomplish a predetermined goal*. Management is a skill that is constantly tested and molded through interpersonal encounters. Its style is determined as much by those who are managed as by the manager. This chapter will address three prominent issues in the management of people in discharge planning: delegation, motivation, and power.

DELEGATION

"Delegation" is a key word in management. That one word represents a clear understanding of roles, a sensitivity to interpersonal relationships and power structures, and the leadership ability to coordinate activities to achieve a goal. If considered superficially, delegation is little more than drawing straws to see who will do what! In discharge planning programs there is a definite need to delegate effectively. Discharge planning includes the patient, the family or significant other persons, the physician, and other health care team members, as well as community resources. As in an orchestra, each performer has a particular role to play, but the performers need both the score and the conductor to avoid total cacophony. If only the conductor has the score, the most magnificent direction will produce only silence.

To manage people is to influence their behavior. If the process is skillful and ethical, the influence is positive. Discharge planning consultants influence the behavior of physicians, hospital staff, patients, families, and community agencies. Behavior is positively influenced by clarifying each individual's goals and objectives, troubleshooting problem areas, delegating responsibilities, coordinating actions, and evaluating results. The tools of discharge planning are the tools of management: assessment and diagnosis of a problem, development and implementation of a plan, and evaluation of the outcome. It is the skill with which these tools are used that reflects the quality of the manager's performance.

For instance, the implementation of a discharge plan will succeed only when all participants know what is expected of them and accept that responsibility. The discharge planning consultant has the responsibility to influence each person's behavior so that roles are understood, accepted, and fulfilled. The irony of the situation is that when participants do not meet their responsibilities, the discharge planning consultant tends to focus on the failure of the others to do their part, rather than on his or her own failure to successfully influence behavior. For example, a referral form must usually accompany a patient on discharge to a nursing home. The consultant works with the primary care nurse to delegate the responsibility for completion of the form to the appropriate disciplines on the health care team—the physician for medical orders, the dietitian for a nutritional history, and so on. If these persons fail to complete their section of the referral, the discharge planning consultant and the primary care nurse bear some of the responsibility. The person responsible for coordinating the discharge planning must be taught to be an *effective* manager.

In discharge planning programs many assumptions are made. It is assumed that discharge planning will begin on admission. It is assumed that the patient and the family will participate in planning for discharge. It is assumed that the discharge planning personnel will assist in the development of a plan that will be carried out by the appropriate agencies or facilities. It is assumed that if everyone cooperates, the plan will work and that the patient will benefit. There are only two assumptions an effective delegator can afford to make: (1) If all participants, including the patient, clearly understand what is expected of them, there is a better chance that they will perform their assigned tasks; and (2) if the individual providers and patient believe that the discharge plan is worthwhile, there is an increased chance that everyone involved will perform well.

The proposed discharge plan should be written and kept in an area that is accessible to *all* participants. The proposed discharge plan should include short- and long-range goals, a list of problems, plans to meet the problems, and a list of responsibilities and the persons *delegated* to carry out the plans. Participants are thus provided with clear "contracts" that can be reinforced daily. In particular, the patient and family should know exactly what their role in the plan is and what they may expect from the health care team. Since the plan is written, the patient and family can respond to the goals and voice their acceptance or rejection at the start. When the discharge plan is not written, they may set different goals from those of the health care team, which would inevitably lead to conflict and failure of the plan. The written plan can also be analyzed later to illustrate possible reasons for success or failure of a particular component. It cannot be assumed that a plan acceptable to all is necessarily the plan that will succeed—it is only more likely to succeed. It also cannot be assumed that delegating responsibilities necessarily means that they will be carried out. There is still the issue of motivation.

MOTIVATION

The way managers deal with a lack of motivation in persons who are crucial to the success of a discharge plan is a prominent issue in discharge planning management. Managers can start with some introspection as to what motivates an individual to do a good job: Money? A pleasant work environment? Self-esteem? Power? Money probably provides enough motivation to go to work every day, and a good work environment makes the work more palatable. However, it is self-esteem and power that actually motivate most people to produce quality work.

Self-esteem is a mirror image. It is unlikely that a person who is not respected by others will achieve self-respect. A manager must provide that mirror. It is important to be sensitive to what effect words and actions have on a person—whether they reinforce or inhibit self-esteem and performance.

Fostering self-esteem is also critical in dealing with patients and families. For example, when Mr. Jones is ill, he and his family may be emotionally drained. Doctors and nurses have stripped him of his clothes, probed his body, and imposed the hospital's schedules and routines on him. Mr. Jones has been told when to eat, when to sleep, when to exercise, when to get out of bed, and even at times when to void. His family has been restricted to visiting hours convenient for the hospital. They have often been told only what the staff wanted them to know—and yet no one seems to understand why the family is reluctant to take on the responsibility of caring for Mr. Jones at home. The hospital staff has robbed the patient and his family of their self-esteem.

Discharge planning consultants can help the staff foster self-esteem by supporting an active role for the patient and the family in the discharge plan. The compliant patient who accepts the staff's plan must no longer be idealized. Instead, primary providers must learn to explore appropriate options with the patient regarding discharge plans and to allow the patient to decide with the family which of these options is personally acceptable. Early discharge planning necessitates the family's involvement and diminishes the chances of their becoming outsiders. It provides them with a specific role to play; they are given responsibilities. The family and the patient should know they have influence over the outcome and thus can develop self-esteem.

The role of each participant in the discharge plan must be determined by individual strengths. If a delegator overestimates a person's capabilities, failure may ensue, because unachievable tasks have been assigned. If a delegator underestimates a person's abilities, interest may be lost, and performance may decline. In either case, self-esteem suffers.

Discharge planning personnel should also capitalize on opportunities to provide positive reinforcement to participants in the discharge plan who have performed well. For example, a written memorandum complimenting a person on a well-written referral, with a copy sent to the supervisor, may be one way to raise self-esteem. Thank-you notes from families and patients should be shared with all participants in the discharge plan. A copy of an exemplary referral or written discharge plan should be put into the employee's record if at all possible as an example of high performance on which performance evaluation can be based. Rewards are important to everyone, and recognizing and implementing appropriate ones should be a high priority for discharge planning personnel who seek to motivate others.

POWER

There are power structures in any organization, and they are not necessarily determined by authority. *Authority is delegated from above; power is bestowed from below*. Discharge planning personnel do not usually possess power by authority. For instance, the discharge planning consultant seldom has direct authority over the nursing staff or physicians. The consultant's power is usually derived from performance and personality. If the consultant consistently performs the assigned role and develops a reputation for competence, then power is more easily acquired. If the competent performance of duties is recognized as also enhancing the performance of others, power is almost assured. In addition, if the consultant possesses personal attributes that are pleasing to others, power is attained.

Demonstration of competence requires that the role of the discharge planning personnel be clearly defined and understood by others. For example, the head nurse on a particular unit may believe that it is the role of the discharge planning personnel to contact a visiting nurse agency with specific orders at the time of the patient's discharge. When the discharge planning consultant consistently requests that the head nurse assign a staff nurse to call the referral in, the head nurse becomes angry. Unless the discharge planning personnel clarify their roles with the head nurse, they may lose the head nurse's respect, and thus the power to influence that nurse is diminished.

To demonstrate competence, discharge planning personnel must be visible. They can function as role models for the nursing staff in the development of management skills, and they can demonstrate accountability for planning that will meet the client's health needs. Discharge planning personnel should learn to view the nursing unit as their office and spend as much time as possible in the mainstream of activity. Only then will the nurse, as well as the patient and other members of the health care team, have sufficient exposure to the discharge planning personnel to develop an understanding and respect for their competence.

Having power is one matter; effectively utilizing it is another. Discharge planning personnel depend on cooperation and the sharing of common goals in preparing a discharge plan. Effective managers recognize, however, that conflicts of interest may arise in any plan. If that conflict is so highly charged as to threaten another's power, cooperation may be impossible to achieve. To be effective, the discharge planning personnel must control conflicts, particularly among persons with the most power, who presumably have the most to lose.

A classic example of controlling power conflicts in discharge planning can be found within the utilization review program. The hospital is concerned with the patient's welfare but must also be concerned with length of stay and cost containment. The physician has the power to admit and discharge patients, but the utilization review committee (URC) controls the Blue Cross and Medicare payments. The patient trusts the physician to know when he is ready for discharge, and the physician stands to lose that trust if the patient receives a 24-hour notice from URC that he must be discharged or be responsible for the hospital bill. (The URC letter states only that the patient's hospital stay will no longer be covered by Medicare or Blue Cross, not that he must be discharged; yet the impact is the same.) If, in addition, the services the patient needs are not immediately available so that he *can* be discharged within 24 hours, both the patient and the physician will become angry, and more often than not the discharge planning program bears the brunt of that anger.

If the discharge planning consultant analyzes the situation, a workable plan can be developed to avoid such conflicts. *Early* discharge planning and a close working relationship with URC is absolutely essential. If at all possible, the discharge planning department should have a representative at the URC meetings to foster mutual understanding of roles and to provide a means of demonstrating competence to the committee. If ongoing dialogue is established, no one should be surprised by discontinuance of insurance benefits letters from URC, and discharge plans should be ready to be implemented. If services are still not available when the patient is ready to be discharged, the discharge planning personnel should know the reason. Anger can then be channeled toward constructive public relations efforts in the community so that the ability to react to the patient's needs after discharge can be improved. Power is then a positive influence. The long-range effect of this effort is a strong public image of the discharge planning department, which constitutes a power base from which the discharge planning program can flourish.

DIRECTING PERSONNEL IN A DISCHARGE PLANNING DEPARTMENT

Directors of discharge planning programs have some special management problems to consider. They include how to effectively staff a discharge planning department, how to effectively lead a discharge planning department, and how to appraise the performance of the discharge planning staff.

Staffing a discharge planning department is difficult for several reasons, one of which is money. Most of the discharge planning departments are not revenue producing, and the discharge planning director will need to compromise to meet budget constraints. Another reason is that there is no one way to staff a discharge planning department. One 300-bed facility may have two staff members in the department; another may have ten. One department may consist entirely of social workers, another of nurses, and still another of representatives of multiple disciplines. Other facilities may split the functions among departments. Directors may find that what was expedient staffing to meet the needs of the institution five to ten years previously is not appropriate in the light of present long-range goals.

One principle that will assist the director in staffing a department is that the authority and responsibility for discharge planning should remain with the primary health care providers. If there seems to be a need to increase discharge planning personnel, the director should first analyze the activities of the department to determine whether it has "assumed" responsibilities that belong elsewhere. If this has occurred, other health care team members must be educated and willing to assume these responsibilities. The director must work closely within their power structures to win concessions here.

Likewise, the director should include discharge planning personnel in planning intradepartmental change and redefining roles, policies, and procedures. Certain tasks may interfere with the activities of the department's personnel, who we will assume for now to be either nurses or social workers. It may not be appropriate, however, for other departments to assume these tasks. Discharge planning directors should consider the use of ancillary personnel within the department to perform these functions. Four distinct types of personnel already utilized in some discharge planning departments are medical advisers, program assistants, financial counselors, and nursing home liaison facilitators.

The medical adviser maintains a liaison between the discharge planning department and the other medical doctors on the staff and in the community. The role is an advisory one and does not replace direct communication between discharge planning personnel and the attending physician. Rather, the medical adviser is an adjunct to the attending physician, attending case conferences for discharge planning and clarifying medical diagnoses and treatment plans for the benefit of the other participants in the plan. The adviser's responsibility is to ensure the continuity of medical care for patients in their discharge planning and also to share in the education of the professionals in the discharge planning program.

Another valuable addition to the department is a program assistant. This person is responsible for educational and administrative functions as well as some secretarial functions. She is responsible for coordinating all unit secretarial roles that directly relate to the discharge planning process—for example, the mailing of referral forms. The statistical data collected for evaluation purposes are also gathered and assembled by the program assistant. If properly prepared for the position, the program assistant can function as a key resource person for physicians, nurses, unit secretaries, and community agencies by providing information and assistance in referral and procedural matters. The program assistant's screening of routine phone messages received by discharge planning personnel should alone substantiate the need for this position in a department; however, she is far more valuable than that single role indicates.

A financial counselor may appropriately work with the family specifically in regard to eligibility for financial assistance after discharge. Business office personnel are primarily concerned with payment of hospital costs and are not usually well versed in coverage for long-term care or home care. Private insurance varies dramatically in available coverage and may even vary among group policies within the same insurance agency. The counselor should maintain close working relationships with such agencies as the department of public welfare, the Social Security Administration, the Veterans Administration, and the Commission for the Blind. Competently prepared applications directed to key personnel within these agencies can substantially reduce time spent waiting for approvals. Having one person in the department who is an expert in this area reduces time spent in educating other personnel in financial matters.

A nursing home liaison facilitator has a unique role in the discharge planning program. The development of such a position is a direct consequence of the increasing shortage of available, acceptable nursing home beds in many areas. Discharge planning personnel must be confident that the program facilitates appropriate placement. This goal can be accomplished only if the facilities utilized are familiar to the department and cooperate with the department's efforts to match patients and facilities. The nursing home liaison facilitator has a public relations role. This employee is in daily contact by phone with most of the facilities routinely utilized and is responsible for finding available beds in appropriate facilities based on the assessment of level of care provided by the discharge planning coordinator. When a facility accepts a patient, the nursing home liaison facilitator reports back to the appropriate discharge planning personnel, who will make the final determination as to its suitability for the patient. This employee also schedules and participates in on-site visits to facilities to gather data on their specific qualities. This information is maintained by the liaison facilitator in written nursing home profiles available to all discharge planning personnel, patients, families, and hospital staff. Departments that have developed such a position generally report favorable reactions by the nursing homes with which they work. The nursing homes have one person to work with at the hospital and find that this arrangement conserves time and effort, increases the quality of communication, and facilitates follow-up.

The nursing home liaison facilitator also compliles statistics regarding patients placed in long-term care facilities, for use by the director of the discharge planning department, the hospital's administrators, and the departments of public welfare and public health. These data are utilized to evaluate trends in the patient population requiring institutionalization and to evaluate the demands this population places on the hospital, the discharge planning department, and the region's resources. Finally, the nursing home liaison facilitator reports routinely to the utilization review committee, listing the patients within the hospital who are awaiting placement in a long-term care facility. This list includes the level of care and special problems inhibiting discharge for each of these patients. The utilization review coordinators utilize this information in considering termination of insurance benefits for continued hospitalization.

The director of a discharge planning department should adopt the same principles of management that are expected of the staff of discharge planning personnel. These principles are as follows:

1. The director should provide a strong role model for discharge planning personnel.
2. The job description of the director should be shared with discharge planning personnel.
3. The director must demonstrate competence as a manager.
4. The director must foster self-esteem in discharge planning personnel.
5. The director should use power effectively.

Performance evaluations can be a means to foster mutual respect. If directors of discharge planning programs are confident in their own competence and believe in the worth of the evaluation process, the evaluation is more likely to be a positive *exchange* of ideas. Confident directors ask employees to evaluate the performance of the director and the department, as well as their own performance. Together goals are set and past objectives are evaluated. The employee shares the responsibility for documenting performance that demonstrates attainment of the goals. The manager's comments should be specific and should reinforce the positive aspects of the employee's performance while inhibiting continuance of negative actions.

It is important that new employees be given written job descriptions that clearly delineate what is expected of them. At the time of evaluation, performance must be measured against these same expectations. Directors of discharge planning departments should also work toward the development of standards of performance that can be utilized in evaluations. Such performance standards must be clear and must be given to the employee prior to evaluation. They are useful only if there is a means of measuring performance against them. If there is no means of documenting performance in the area of follow-up, it will be difficult to assess how well the employee is performing within the standards given.

Directors should meet with employees weekly for supervision if at all possible. An annual evaluation should be a summary of the ongoing evaluations that occurred all year. Staff meetings should be held for the purposes of collectively evaluating the department's performance, developing department objectives, and solving problems. Individual supervision and staff meetings should include discussion and recognition of successes as well as problems so that "gripe sessions" can be avoided. If performance evaluations are successfully implemented, both the employees and the manager will learn to look forward to them. Such meetings can provide a time to stop and catch one's breath, pat oneself on the back for past achievements, and forge ahead on a new path.

SUMMARY

In summary, discharge planning is a process that is successful only if it is skillfully directed. The responsibility for discharge planning belongs on the front line with the direct health care providers and the patient. The direction of that planning belongs in the hands of the managers. The director of the discharge planning department, the discharge planning personnel, and the discharge planning coordinator on the patient care unit are all managers; their actions affect the performance of others. If they are good managers, their actions will have a positive influence. In either case, they cannot escape the fact that their role is to manage. Once this is recognized and accepted, the structure of the discharge planning program comes into clearer focus. Each program will have its own needs, priorities, and restrictions, but sound management practices can be implemented usually without widespread changes in organization. As long as two or more persons are involved in the discharge plan, there will be a need for effective delegation, motivation, and use of power. Effective management is not "frosting." It is the basic ingredient in a successful program.

ACKNOWLEDGMENT

We would like to thank Diane Ricca for the assistance she gave to this chapter by sharing the role she created and implemented as Program Assistant in the Continuing Care Program at Boston Hospital for Women.

ADDITIONAL READINGS

Douglass, L. M., and Bevis, E. O.: Nursing management and leadership in action: principles and applications to staff situations, ed. 3, St. Louis, 1979, The C. V. Mosby Co.

Stone, S., Berger, M. S., Elhart, D., et al., editors: Management for nurses: a multidisciplinary approach, St. Louis, 1976, The C. V. Mosby Co.

Thompson, D. W.: Managing people: influencing behavior, St. Louis, 1978, The C. V. Mosby Co.

CHAPTER 7

Management of multidisciplinary communication in discharge planning

KATHLEEN M. McKEEHAN
CYNTHIA MacDONALD WALSH
JANET PAPILE O'DAY

Many years ago, mystics of Zen Buddhism posed a riddle that asks, "Is there a sound in the forest if a tree crashes down and no one is around to hear it?" The answer to the riddle is no, there is no sound unless someone hears it. This same analogy can be applied to the process of communication. There must be someone who receives (as in sound or touch), or there is no communication. Communication is defined as the *process of passing information and understanding from one person to another.*[2] Multidisciplinary communication is the insertion of persons from various disciplines into that process. According to Rubin and associates,[7] delivery of health care—as opposed to just the delivery of medical care, nursing care, or social care—always involves a team of persons from multiple disciplines. This chapter will offer insights into patterns of multidisciplinary communication. We will analyze how the communication modes among disciplines and between disciplines often enhance or impede the discharge planning process.

CURRENT MODES OF MULTIDISCIPLINARY COMMUNICATION

Peter Drucker, well known in the field of management, once stated: "The communication gap within institutions and between groups in society has been widening steadily—to the point where it threatens to become an unbridgeable gulf of total misunderstanding. Yet, there is an information explosion."[3] In the field of management a distinction has been drawn between information and communication. Information is referred to as impersonal data free from the human component, whereas communication has human emotion and values. Many workers in the area of discharge planning have been frustrated by the imbalance between the information explosion and communication gaps—communication gaps that exist both within the institution's multidisciplinary departments and between the institution and community resources.

There are two major modes of multidisciplinary communcation: formal and informal. Both modes may be transmitted by oral or written means.

Formal multidisciplinary communication

To understand formal lines of multidisciplinary communication, one must first understand the organizational structure in health care facilities (whether they be hospitals or nursing homes). According to Longest,[6] a noted author on the subject of management practices in health care, the organizational structure located within health care facilities is quite different from the typical "bureaucratic pyramid" found in industry (Fig. 7-1). He refers to the structure in health care facilities as the "dual pyramid" (Fig. 7-2). Longest further states that the difference results from the unusual relationship between the formal authority represented by the administrative hierarchy and the authority of knowledge passed by health professionals in the hospital. With regard to discharge planning policies, the formal lines of communication might encompass multiple pyramids involving the hierarchy in every multidisciplinary department in the facility, including the professional standards review organization (PSRO) (Fig. 7-3). Thus, one goal of every discharge planning program should be to gain an awareness of *all* the facility's policies, procedures, and authority structure that relate to discharge planning. This awareness is a necessity if a discharge planning program is to be instrumental in bridging communication gaps both within the facility and between the facility and the community.

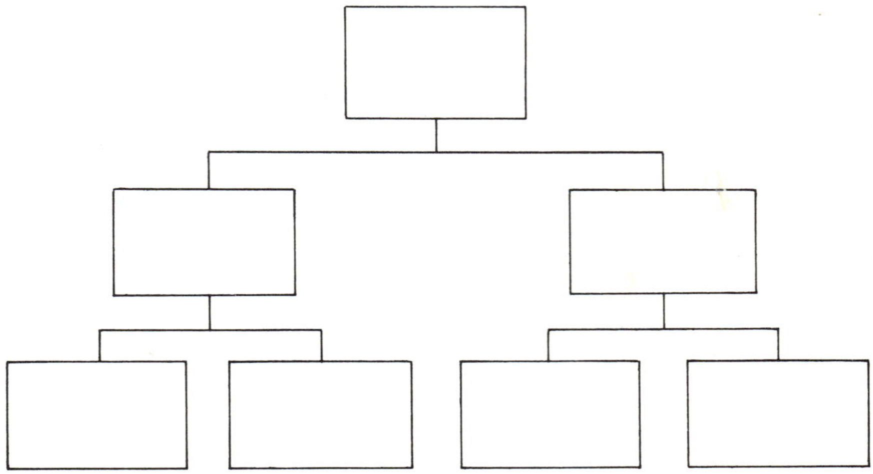

Fig. 7-1. Typical bureaucratic pyramid.

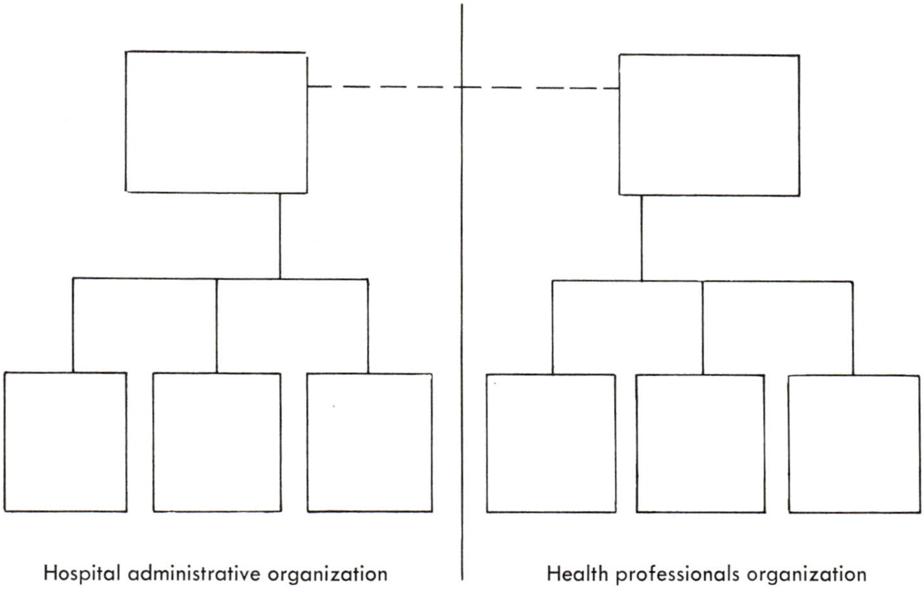

Fig. 7-2. Dual pyramid of typical hospital.

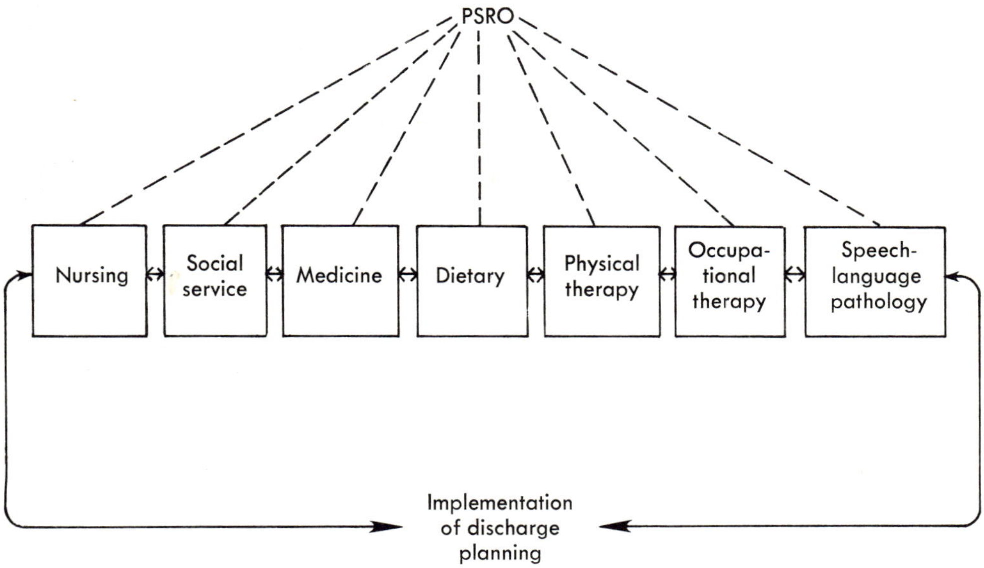

Fig. 7-3. Organizational framework for multidisciplinary communication. The arrows are multidimensional: each department can communicate directly with the others.

Informal multidisciplinary communication

Informal communication is often referred to as the grapevine. Evidence in management research shows that over 80% of grapevine information is accurate; however, even though it is accurate, it often has missing components, which may lead to misinterpretation.[2] Evidence further shows that the grapevine is influential, either in a favorable or an unfavorable way. The point to be made here is that discharge planning program personnel need to examine the informal communications mode within their facility, learn the patterns of the grapevine, and seek to influence it. Keith Davis, a noted author on human behavior, summarized the importance of the grapevine in the following way:

> The object is to get this vine to bear desirable fruit—to integrate its interests with those of the formal organization. Managers today are getting on the grapevine in order to learn who its leaders are, how it operates, and what information it carries. Then they attempt to "feed, water, and cultivate the grapevine." Facts are fed into it so that motivation for rumormongering is reduced. . . . The grapevine in some ways benefits the organization.[2]

Within your institution there may be disciplines in which there is particular interest in the aftercare of patients. This interest can be used to build the base of the discharge planning program. For example, if there are a few physicians who are particularly good in the discharge planning process, speak through them to other physicians at staff meetings. If there are particular nurses, social workers, and others who work creatively with patients and staff in discharge planning, point them out as examples for persons in their own disciplines to model. It is important to state here that every facility has at least one particular person who is constantly involved both in formal and informal communication regarding discharge planning. That person is the utilization review or PSRO coordinator. This coordinator examines the admission and discharge practices of every physician on the staff and is frequently found "where the action is," that is, on the units, reading and rereading patient progress notes. It is important for discharge planning personnel to have close, continuous communication with this coordinator.

After analyzing the formal and informal mutlidisciplinary communications systems within a facility setting, it is important for the discharge planning personnel to define specific goals regarding current communication patterns. It is these goals and the objectives created to attain them that can break down the territorial barriers that often impede quality discharge planning.

PRINCIPLES RELATED TO TEAMWORK

According to Rubin and associates,[7] a team is a group with a specified task, the accomplishment of which requires the interdependent and collaborative efforts of its members. Teamwork is a core component within every discharge planning program. For this reason there should be formal goals and objectives that speak to the enhancement of multidisciplinary communication in teamwork. An example of a general goal might be *the creation of a multidisciplinary team approach in the discharge planning process of this facility*. An example of an objective to attain that goal might be *to establish multidisciplinary team rounds on every unit at a specified time for the purpose of discussing the discharge planning of patients with primary providers of care*.

It is interesting to note that little energy is given to formally educating persons from various disciplines to work together and communicate as a team. Often educational strategy subverts managerial strategy. For example, members of each discipline are educated in separate professional schools. Then, after graduation, each professional is expected to press an invisible button and magically know how to work with others on a team in the delivery of health care. The results, as many persons know, can be disastrous. Because there is a lack of knowledge of the various roles played in the delivery of health care, strict territorial barriers are often erected that impede team development and ultimately interfere with quality patient care. This is not to deny that certain professional territories are important for legal reasons. The point emphasized here is that we should maximize rather than minimize what is taught in team settings and provide an environment in which members of various disciplines can learn together and have the opportunity to be educated in the process of teamwork.

According to sociologist J. W. Eaton, there are three major issues that have important implications in the management of teams:

1. The effects of different backgrounds and "reference groups" on collaborative work.
   When people from different backgrounds are asked to work as colleagues or peers a lot of tension may be produced. For example, an internist trained to a doctor-patient relationship may have real difficulty in "sharing" the patient.
2. The effects of "professionalism" on carrying out the work.
   Any organization composed of a variety of capabilities always faces an issue of multiple loyalties: loyalties to the organization, loyalties to the task, and loyalties to the profession.
3. The effects of changing and different value systems on the people and the work.
   Multiple value systems of both patient populations and providers of care should be taken into consideration.[4]

Some educational institutions have faced the problem of territorial barriers by offering formal multidisciplinary courses in delivery of health care. A good example of such a course is one offered at the University of Colorado Medical Center. The course is entitled "Health Professionals, Health Issues, and Family Study" and is offered to both medical students and nursing students together. A major objective of the course is to acquaint a member of one health profession with a member of another health profession and to clarify through interaction one another's roles, goals, and approaches to patient care. This objective is accomplished in two ways: didactically in the classroom, and empirically with families in the community. The University of Colorado is to be commended for taking the risk to teach "reality."

In a recent article in *Hospitals*, Richard Edwards states that "professionals in alliance achieve more effective discharge planning."[5] Professional alliance is described as nonterritorial, complementary roles of interacting professionals working together for the achievement of responsible and responsive discharge planning with patients. It takes persons who are mature and secure in their roles to work as colleagues in health care teams. The name of the game is trust and mutual respect: trusting that each member of each discipline is a caring, competent provider of health care, and respecting the distinctive body of knowledge encompassed in the role of each discipline.

STRATEGIES FOR IMPLEMENTING MULTIDISCIPLINARY COMMUNICATION IN DISCHARGE PLANNING

Health care teams evolve in two ways: informally by chance, or formally for the purpose of attaining a specific good. Discharge planning programs have the distinct opportunity of formally creating teams of individuals from multiple disciplines with the defined purpose of enhancing the planning and delivery of comprehensive, family-centered health care. As stated before, the discharge planning department acts as a consultant group to primary providers. Because of the traditional pattern of educating members of different disciplines on a separatist model, the following specific strategies are often necessary to enhance the quality of multidisciplinary communication within health care teams.

General factors affecting multidisciplinary team meetings

Multidisciplinary team meetings can be productive; however, their productivity rests on four major ingredients: structure, product, leadership, and climate.

Structure involves such components as the physical setting, the size of the group, the agenda, the frequency of meetings, and the promptness and length of meetings. All team meetings should be held in a quiet physical setting devoid of interruptions. The size of the group should be kept to a manageable number; the literature has suggested six to eight participants.[1] An agenda is an effective tool for organization. It is an imperative ingredient if the meeting is to achieve its purpose. Agendas should be distributed ahead of the meeting to allow the members time to prepare for their participation. Consistency of meeting times helps members arrange their calendars for future attendance. Every person's time should be considered as valuable; therefore meetings should start promptly and end as scheduled. There should be adequate physical space and appropriate temperature control. Round tables are more conducive to communication than square tables.

The *product* of multidisciplinary team meetings usually involves three factors: the purpose of the meeting, the preparation for the meeting, and follow-up of the results of the meeting. The purpose of the meeting should be defined and stated clearly to all members. Preparation for the meeting is enhanced when relevant information is given to team members before the actual meeting takes place. Follow-up on the results of specific team discussions offers a means of evaluating plans of care. It also offers a "stroking" mechanism to reward individuals for their involvement.

Leadership in team meetings is important; it often spells their success or failure. Democratic leadership is the most effective style for most multidisciplinary team meetings, but a temporary switch to an autocratic style may be necessary to control individuals exhibiting inappropriate behavior.

Climate refers to the human factors involved in team meetings, such as free exchange of information, feelings of members, or the existence of cliques. Open discussion tends to foster effective meetings. Feelings of being relaxed usually correlate with an understanding of the purpose of the meeting and a familiarity with the members and their roles. Cliques have been defined as "small, exclusive circles of people." They sometimes can be disruptive, as when private conversations are carried on during the meeting while other persons are talking. Temporary autocratic leadership may help everyone to return to the meeting's focus.

There are two major types of multidisciplinary team meetings directly involved in the discharge planning process: rounds, and predischarge and postdischarge planning conferences. They differ from each other in the following way: Rounds are an activity in which individuals meet to *review* the current status of numerous patients on a particular unit. Most medical personnel are familiar with the terms "medical rounds," "nursing rounds," and "social service rounds." Predischarge and postdischarge planning conferences are formal multidisciplinary meetings held to create and implement discharge plans with specific patients. The meetings usually involve discussions of patients with multiple complex needs.

Rounds

Since many facilities already have a set of rounds in operation, it is often beneficial to assimilate discharge planning into the existing rounds. One advantage of this approach is that it could eliminate another committee meeting. Since staff time is often limited, the last thing needed is another committee meeting that will reduce time available for patient care. Discharge planning should fit into existing priorities; however, at the same time the staff may need to be educated to raise discharge planning to a high priority within the delivery of health care. This educational process is lengthy, but it is definitely achievable. For those facilities that lag behind, discharge planning has already been encompassed within JCAH and PSRO regulations. The push to prioritize discharge planning will soon be mandatory.

There are three major factors that are important for successful rounds involving discharge planning. First, rounds should be *multidisciplinary,* with representation from those disciplines primarily involved in the delivery of care on a specific unit. Second, they should be held at a *consistent* time of the day and frequently enough to allow for the discussion of at least 75% of all patient discharges. (This does not mean that 75% of all patients must be discussed. It simply means that rounds should occur often enough during one week so that there will be an opportunity to discuss patients before 75% are discharged.) Third, they should be held in an area and at a time as *devoid of interruptions* as possible. A quiet place away from the business of the day's activities could be used, or "walking rounds" that would enhance patient participation in discharge planning could be held.

The key to successful multidisciplinary discharge planning rounds is flexibility. If an emergency occurs on the floor, rounds could be held later in the day or the next day. If a specific member cannot attend rounds, they should take place anyway. Rounds should not be built around a specific discipline; they should be built around patient needs and the matching of services to fulfill those needs.

Predischarge and postdischarge planning conferences

As previously defined, predischarge and postdischarge planning conferences are formal, multidisciplinary meetings held to create and implement discharge plans with specific patients. Important factors that spell their success are threefold. First, they must involve the patient and significant other persons either directly or indirectly. The best plan is sure to fail without a commitment to the plan by the patient and the significant others in his life. Second, the conferences should include appropriate multidisciplinary primary providers and consultants both from within the facility and representing community agencies. Attendance by appropriate individuals will save hours of valuable time spent tracking them down to validate information. Third, the conferences should be scheduled during a specified time that is convenient for all persons and that is suitable in relation to the patient's continuum of care. As an illustration of fitting into that continuum of care, a predischarge conference could be held early enough during a patient's hospital stay so that discharge plans can be comfortably carried out. As another example, a conference could be held after discharge, when the patient has been involved with the community agency long enough to test specific approaches to plans of care. It is important to point out here that postdischarge conferences provide an excellent opportunity for follow-up and evaluation of patient care plans. They also offer a support mechanism to individuals in community resource agencies, who tend at times to feel isolated from the discharge planning process.

Facility policies and procedures affecting multidisciplinary communication

One strategy to enhance multidisciplinary communication that should be basic to all discharge planning programs is the inclusion of a multidisciplinary approach in all policies and procedures. A good example would be a specific written procedure for processing a referral to a visiting nurse association. This procedure should provide guidelines for all the disciplines to follow as they implement their role in completing the referral form.

An example of a policy that affects discharge planning would be the integration of discharge planning into the format utilized for patient histories and assessment forms, such as medical histories, nursing assessments, and other multidisciplinary information forms. If we truly believe in the philosophy that discharge planning begins at the moment of the patient's admission, then one way to implement that philosophy is to include a discharge planning component on all initial patient information intake sheets.

For many facilities the nursing Kardex is the major vehicle used in passing pertinent patient information from shift to shift and from discipline to discipline. Since nurses provide the most consistent 24-hour care to patients, they are usually the primary coordinators of the discharge planning process. Discharge planning information should be available on all Kardex systems. Some facilities choose to categorize this information through the use of a "discharge planning checklist" or a written discharge plan at the patient's bedside.

In-service education orientation programs

Another strategy for implementing multidisciplinary communication within the discharge planning process is to include principles of discharge planning within every discipline's orientation program. Actions often speak louder than words; therefore one of the best ways to utilize this strategy is to have various disciplines actually participate in the orientation of other disciplines. For example, social workers, dietitians, and physical therapists might actively participate in a nursing in-service program on discharge planning. This approach would allow members of each discipline to directly relate their role of primary provider or consultant to the discharge planning process.

Presentations at departmental management meetings

Every multidisciplinary department has regular management meetings. Examples of these meetings include medical staff meetings, head nurse and supervisor meetings, and social service departmental meetings. It is imperative that the discharge planning process be on the agenda at these meetings *at least* annually. One way to be included on the agenda is for the discharge planning personnel to ask whether they might discuss their annual report for the purpose of including the specific department's suggestions in the future year's goals for the discharge planning program. It is crucial that discharge planning personnel hear suggestions directly and regularly, so that needed changes can be made to ensure development.

Newsletters and memorandums

Another successful strategy for implementing multidisciplinary communication is the creative use of vehicles of communication already existent within a facility or community, such as a monthly newsletter or periodic memorandums disseminated throughout the departments. There is no faster way of gaining attention than placing people in print. One hospital wrote a delightful true story about the discharge of a patient known to almost everyone in the institution. The story depicted the discharge planning process step by step, outlining the roles of each involved discipline. The story provided an opportunity for the discharge planning program to achieve multiple objectives. First, the institution was provided with an illustrated explanation of what the discharge planning program is and how it facilitates the discharge planning process. Second, members of specific disciplines were offered an opportunity to understand activities of other disciplines depicted in the story. Third, a feedback mechanism was provided for patients and community resource agencies to speak directly to the staff through the story. The fourth objective was strictly educational. It was reached in the summary of the story, where the author spoke directly to the do's and don'ts of discharge planning.

Memorandums are a good example of a direct educational mechanism. They provide a vehicle for dissemination of information to all departments and are the fastest way to inform departments of problems, successes, or changes in the discharge planning program. It is important to remember that since many other departments use memorandums as their sole vehicle of communication, recipients may become desensitized to their contents. Follow-up on all memorandums to validate their effectiveness is therefore necessary.

Representation on community advisory committees

One of the best ways of affecting multidisciplinary lines of communication between a facility and the community is through representation on community agency advisory committees. In this day and age almost every community agency has an advisory committee. It is important that every facility allocate time for discharge planning personnel to attend community advisory committee meetings. Since "time is money," this opportunity could be priceless in providing benefits to both the facility and the community agency. Depending on a specific committee's power and influence in overall policy management, a potential exists that may greatly affect the quality of discharge planning.

Multidisciplinary referral form

The most important vehicle of multidisciplinary communication in the entire discharge planning process is the *referral form.* The essential components of a referral form were discussed in detail in Chapter 1. It is important to reemphasize here that discharge planning personnel must continue to be aware of the work being done nationally in the area of patient assessment for purpose of referral. The annotated bibliography (Appendix A) offers a section in which references specifically related to referral forms are marked with an asterisk.

In many ways the referral form is analogous to a photograph of the patient. It depicts all the special areas that make the patient and his health status unique. Just as no other medium has the ability to depict "reality" more vividly than photography, nothing else has the ability to affect the provision of the continuing care of patients more decisively than the referral form. Continuing the analogy between photography and referral form writing, there are four ingredients that are imperative to both for a successful product. First, just as a photograph depicts a specific subject, the referral form should be patient oriented. Second, a photograph shows things as they are; the referral form should be objective in its assessment but should offer an opportunity for providers to suggest a plan of care. Third, a photograph has the ability to depict its subject from various angles; the referral form should have a multidisciplinary approach. Fourth, a photograph can be used in various settings (e.g., newspapers and museums); the referral form should encompass information for home care agencies as well as facility placement.

Unfortunately, one of the major problems in most discharge planning programs is a poor referral form. The picture of the patient may be so blurred that the receiving agency may not even be able to recognize who the patient is, much less know how to proceed with care. If health providers truly believe that patients have a right to quality discharge planning, then health providers must commit themselves to the development and utilization of appropriate multidisciplinary referral forms.

SUMMARY

In summation, management of multidisciplinary communication is the third component completing the "management practice model" for discharge planning. The essential elements within this component are the current modes of multidisciplinary communication; principles related to teamwork; and strategies for implementing multidisciplinary communication. The patient care referral form is the channel through which multidisciplinary information flows, linking the facility with the community.

REFERENCES

1. Bales, R.: In conference, Harvard Bus. Rev. **32**:44-50, 1954.
2. Davis, K.: Human behavior at work—human relations and organizational behavior, ed. 4, New York, 1972, McGraw-Hill Book Co.
3. Drucker, P. F.: Management: tasks—responsibilities—practices, New York, 1974, Harper & Row, Publishers.
4. Eaton, J. W.: Social processes of professional teamwork, Am. Sociol. **16**:707-713, 1951.
5. Edwards, R. C.: Professionals in "alliance" achieve more effective discharge planning, Hospitals **52**:71, 1978.
6. Longest, B. B.: Management practices for the health professional, Reston, Va., 1976, Reston Publishing Co.
7. Rubin, I., Plovnick, M., and Fry, R.: Improving the coordination of care: a program for health team development, Cambridge, Mass., 1975, Ballinger Publishing Co.

ADDITIONAL READINGS

Hogg, S., Hughes, A., McKeehan, K., and Tucker, G.: Team meetings. Unpublished paper presented to students of management skills in primary health care, Harvard University School of Public Health, Boston, Mass., May 27, 1976.

Rubin, I., Fry, R., and Plovnick, M.: Managing human resources in health care organizations: an applied approach, Reston, Va., 1978, Reston Publishing Co.

SECTION THREE

Implementation of the discharge planning process

This section is the pinnacle of the book. All previous chapters were intended to provide a foundation in preparation for this component. The purpose of this section is to offer the reader an opportunity to examine the roles of individuals from various disciplines as they integrate discharge planning into the delivery of their health care. Role identification is an important educational tool in the mechanism of change. Edgar Schein speaks to this issue when he states: "If the change goal is the acceptance of a particular set of behaviors and attitudes, the change agent should attempt to produce a setting conducive to positive identification and provide the target with a good representation of the point of view to be learned."[1]

In many of the following chapters, you will find examples of forms that have been found useful in patient assessment by a practitioner from a specific discipline. It should be emphasized here that the presence of these forms in no way departs from the philosophy stated in Chapter 1 of the importance of creating an *integrated* referral form with a multidisciplinary approach. The forms presented throughout this section are useful primarily as predischarge assessment guides. They are an adjunct to an integrated referral form that provides a multidisciplinary approach. It is strongly suggested that the reader examine existing referral forms that have undergone significant research. Published data concerning forms already tested are discussed in Chapter 1, and articles related to referral form research and construction are listed in the annotated bibliography (Appendix A) and marked with an asterisk.

REFERENCE

1. From Schein, E. H.: The mechanisms of change. In Bennis, W., and Chin, R., editors: The planning of change, ed. 2, New York, 1969, Holt, Rinehart and Winston, p. 107.

CHAPTER 8

Discharge planning: a staff nurse's perspective

LUCY FEILD

ROLE OF STAFF NURSE IN DISCHARGE PLANNING

Focus of nursing's concern

Hospitalization is for most patients a temporary circumstance in which eventual discharge is a relative certainty. However, intervening factors related to either the cause of admission or the course of hospitalization may significantly alter the patient's ability to resume previous life patterns or functional levels. To ensure that these alterations are identified and provided for in the process of assisting the patient toward an optimum level of wellness, health care providers have a serious responsibility to incorporate formal discharge planning into the delivery of health services.

Every patient has a right to discharge planning, and every member of the health care team has a corresponding responsibility to systematically assess and plan for discharge needs, both immediate and long-term, as a component of care delivery. Specific responsibilities for discharge planning will depend on the role of each discipline in the care of the individual patient, based on the patient's needs.

According to the current system of health care delivery in most sectors, every patient receives some form of nursing care, although the specific nature and amount of this care may vary considerably. The patient is recognized by all health care providers as the focus of care, but each group has a special area of concern. Nursing's special concern, according to Dorothea Orem, is "man's need for self-care action and the provision and management of it on a continuous basis in order to sustain life and health, recover from disease or injury, and cope with their effects."[5,pp.1-2] Orem defines self-care as "the practice of activities that individuals personally initiate and perform on their own behalf in maintaining life, health, and well-being."[5,p.13] A requirement for nursing care occurs when the patient's ability to carry out self-care activities is compromised.

Nursing's advantages in the discharge planning process

As the only discipline on the health care team that is routinely and immediately available to every patient and family on a 24-hour basis, nursing is in a unique position to provide the crucial coordinating link between the patient and all involved disciplines. Inherent in such a role are both advantages and responsibilities.

The physician focuses primarily on the diagnosis and treatment of disease. The nurse, in contrast, is primarily concerned with the patient's ability to cope with and adapt to the physical, psychological, and social changes resulting from illness. The nurse assesses the effect of disease on the patient's ability to carry out self-care activities and then plans appropriate interventions when self-care deficits are determined. Those deficits that will persist after discharge indicate the need for special planning, including multidisciplinary coordination in many cases, to ensure that the patient's self-care requirements continue to be met.

The nurse, situated in the same environment as the patient, is usually in the best position to consistently interact with members of other disciplines involved in the patient's care. This convenient circumstance maximizes the nurse's ability to facilitate communication and cooperative planning among health care team members, in regard to both inpatient activities and discharge planning.

Because the scope of nursing's concern is holistic, the nurse will frequently be the one to identify *less obvious* problems that require intervention by another discipline. Few health care providers would miss the need for a physical therapy consultation for a hemiplegic patient who has suffered a recent stroke, or the urgency of a nutrition consultation for a severely malnourished postsurgical patient. It is the nurse, however, who will probably first identify the slow but progressive loss of muscle strength in a bedridden patient with reduced activity tolerance, or the knowledge deficit regarding minimum daily nutrition requirements exhibited by a young mother whose child has been admitted to the pediatric unit with a diagnosis that has few obvious nutritional implications. In these latter situations the nurse's skills help to identify the need for collaboration with another discipline for problems that, if untreated, could potentially delay discharge or interfere with the patient's attainment of an optimum level of health and function.

The nurse has an excellent opportunity to establish trust-based relationships with patients and their significant other persons as a result of frequent and consistent interpersonal actions. This is particularly true for the nurse on the evening shift, who may be the only professional staff member with whom the patient's family and friends have contact. In such circumstances the nurse can provide the link necessary to include significant others in discharge planning.

The nurse is also in a position to make close observations of psychobehavioral patient responses within the context of time. Data collected at night and on weekends, when few other disciplines are readily available, may significantly affect discharge planning. For example, the patient who becomes confused or incontinent only at night, or the patient who regresses or withdraws when social activity slackens, may require special planning not otherwise identified.

Nursing's responsibilities in the discharge planning process

Several nursing responsibilities are inherent in the discharge planning process:

1. The nurse shares an obligation with other health care team members to promote the provision of the highest possible quality of health care to the patient and family. Patient advocacy is inherent in this responsibility. The ability to function comfortably in such a context should facilitate the nurse's efforts to include the patient in discharge planning and to prevent or resolve possible conflicts when the patient's goals differ from those of the health care team.

2. The nurse must be aware of the available resources for patient care that exist both within the health care facility and in the community, so that patient needs can be matched with these resources when indicated and when desired by the patient. This responsibility requires a thorough understanding of services offered. It is unrealistic to expect the generalist to be cognizant of all community and institutional resources, particularly regarding specific patient populations. The continuing care consultant should be especially valuable as a source of information and liaison facilitator for such a nurse.

3. If discharge planning is to be successful, the nurse must establish and maintain collegial relationships with members of other health care disciplines. These relationships must be based on mutual recognition of, and respect for, each group's unique and necessary contribution to the patient's well-being. When an atmosphere that fosters cooperative teamwork and open communication is developed, the entire process will be facilitated, to the benefit of both the patient and the team.

4. Perhaps most importantly, the nurse must develop a clear concept of the roles and responsibilities inherent in professional nursing. Such an understanding must be accompanied by a willingness to accept accountability for the outcomes of nursing action, so that the potential offered by the nurse's position to help patients attain a maximum level of health and function is achieved. This begins with the nurse's acceptance of *individual* responsibility for discharge planning for specific patients, which must be done whether the mode of care delivery is through functional, team, or primary nursing.

To illustrate this last point, particularly for the benefit of other disciplines, the staff nurse's role in discharge planning will be discussed within the framework of the Standards of Nursing Practice established by the American Nurses' Association in 1973.[1]

DISCHARGE PLANNING PROCESS WITHIN THE FRAMEWORK OF THE ANA STANDARDS OF NURSING PRACTICE

The general purpose of the Standards of Nursing Practice is to provide guidelines for the practice of nursing to ensure quality nursing care delivery to the client/patient. More specifically, the standards "focus on practice, project the nursing process as a systematic approach to nursing care, and provide a means for assessing the quality of nursing care,"[7] emphasizing individual accountability for practice within the context of the client-provider relationship.

If the Standards of Nursing Practice were fully implemented in all practice settings, the problems frequently encountered by the nurse in discharge planning would not be so great. The primary responsibility for implementation of the standards falls to each individual nurse, who must assume responsibility for application to practice.

The standards reflect the nursing process, which includes the problem-solving steps of assessment, diagnosis, prescription, implementation, and evaluation. Consideration of each of the eight standards illustrates how application to practice builds in discharge planning as an inescapable component of nursing care for every patient.

Standard I: *The collection of data about the health status of the client/patient is systematic and continuous. The data are accessible, communicated, and recorded.**

If the nurse is responsible for the diagnosis and treatment of human responses to actual or potential health problems as outlined in numerous nurse practice acts,[2] then the data for such decision making must be both appropriate and adequate. Although the nurse must take into consideration the data collected by other disciplines, such information is usually insufficient to carry out nursing practice at the level expected by the profession. Unfortunately, in many instances, further nursing data are either not collected or are gathered informally and not documented. Although numerous significant factors contribute to this situation, including staffing shortages, organizational structures, priority determinations, and individual values and skill competencies, such reality-based deterrents must continue to be addressed by nursing leaders until viable solutions are found. Inefficient patterns of data collection neglect a basic nursing responsibility and increase the potential for missing problems that must be considered in discharge planning.

The initial data must be collected in an organized and systematic manner as soon as possible after admission, hopefully within the first 24 hours. Assessment continues throughout admission as the patient's condition changes and new data become available.

Because nursing's perspective is holistic, the nursing data base must reflect this scope. Carol Soares's four orders of nursing problems,[6] which include the biophysical, cognitive-perceptual, psychosocial, and cultural-existential realms, provide a framework for assessment.

Biophysical realm. Assessment of functional status on admission helps to identify problems and predict priorities in discharge planning. Comparison of these

---

*Standards are from *Standards of Nursing Practice,* Kansas City, Mo., 1973, American Nurses' Association. Reprinted with permission.

data with current status as discharge nears facilitates progress evaluation and pinpoints specific discharge needs.

Major functional patterns of concern to the nurse include breathing, comfort, communication, elimination, hygiene/grooming/skin integrity, mobility/safety, nutrition, sensory perception, sexuality, and sleep/rest.

Specific assessment questions depend on multiple variables such as the patient's health problems and age. In general, if the nurse's concern is with the patient's ability to carry out self-care activity, initial and subsequent assessments focus on the following areas:

1. How did the patient carry out these functions prior to admission? What assistance (persons, equipment, etc.) was required?
2. In what way and to what extent has the patient's health condition affected current ability to carry out these activities?
3. If deficits exist, what needs for assistance are anticipated, both during hospitalization and after discharge? What resources are available?

Cognitive-perceptual realm. Patient teaching is a major nursing responsibility. The goal of such activity is to ensure that the patient possesses sufficient knowledge and skills regarding individual health conditions and care regimens so that responsibility for self-care after discharge can be safely assumed. General assessment areas include the following:

1. What is the patient's understanding of the health condition? What does this individiual *want* to know and *need* to know?
2. What is the patient's level of readiness to learn? What variables exist that enhance or inhibit learning?
3. What problem-solving and learning skills does the patient exhibit?
4. What resources for learning are available to the patient?

Psychosocial realm. The stress of illness and hospitalization evokes a psychological response of varying degrees in both patients and their significant others. Thus it is essential that the nurse consider this area for the purpose of determining actual or potential problems that suggest the need for prevention or intervention. It is also important to recognize that hospitalization may be only one of many concurrent problems with which the patient must cope. Awareness of how the patient's health situation interfaces with other events and stresses not only helps one to see the situation more clearly from the patient's perspective but also provides information that must be considered in discharge planning. General areas of concern include the following:

1. What are the patient's primary support systems? How available are they?
2. What are the patient's usual patterns of coping with stress? How are these patterns being used to cope with the stress of the current illness?
3. What are the patient's predominant concerns?
4. Are there stresses or events other than illness in the patient's life which are of concern?

5. What is the emotional response of the patient and his significant others to the current health problem?
6. How has illness affected the dynamics of the patient's significant relationships?
7. How has illness affected the patient's self-concept in regard to body image, role performance perception, self-esteem, and personal identity?

Cultural-existential realm. This category reflects concern for higher levels of human functioning and affects all others. The implications for discharge planning are clear. Nursing's concern focuses on the following areas:

1. What are the patient's goals? How has illness affected them?
2. To what does the patient ascribe meaning and value in life? How has illness affected these factors?
3. What are the patient's predominant beliefs regarding health and illness? How do these beliefs affect the patient's response to illness?
4. What cultural and religious beliefs, values, and practices are important to the patient and must be considered in planning for discharge?

Once collected, appropriate data are documented in the patient's record, with due consideration given to confidentiality.

Standard II: *Nursing diagnoses are derived from health status data.*

"Nursing diagnosis" is a relatively new term that describes the familiar judgment activity involved in problem identification. Gordon offers the following definition: "Nursing diagnoses, or clinical diagnoses made by professional nurses, describe actual or potential health problems which nurses, by virtue of their education and experience, are capable and licensed to treat."[4]

Whereas the diagnostic *process* used in problem solving is common to all disciplines, the *content* will vary according to each group's unique focus. Nurses acquire the authority to diagnose and treat patient problems that fall within the realm of professional nursing practice as a result of competence (gained through education and experience) and accountability (mandated through licensure, professional standards, and job responsibility). This authority implies that one can, within the limits of professional domain,

- Gather the necessary data base
- Prescribe *definitive* therapy
- Be held accountable for the outcomes of therapy

Considered within this context, and in light of the focus of nursing's concern, it becomes clear that there is a significant difference between nursing diagnosis and medical diagnosis. Nurses do not make medical diagnoses because they cannot gather the necessary data base, prescribe definitive therapy, and be held primarily accountable for the related outcomes of medical problems. However, in no way does the use of the term "nursing diagnosis" negate the importance of nursing collaboration in the *management* of those diagnoses made by the members of other disciplines. Nurses share a vital responsibility for the management of medical diagnoses through observation and reporting of the patient's condition and response to therapy, through prevention and detection of complications, and through implementation of those parts of the medical regimen that the patient cannot carry out independently.

For example, nursing assessment of a 56-year-old man admitted with a medical diagnosis of diabetes mellitus might result in the following nursing diagnoses:

- *Self-care deficit:* bathing and toileting, related to weakness
- *Knowledge deficit:* medication, diet, activity, and disease process, related to lack of previous instruction
- *Alteration in self-concept,* related to perceived implications of diabetes

The physician is responsible for designing a therapeutic regimen to manage the diabetes. The nurse, on the other hand, will assist the patient with the self-care activities he cannot do for himself, teach him about the disease process and its management within the context of his life-style, and help him begin to accept and cope with the fact that he is diabetic. Appropriate collaborative nursing responsibilities include observation, preventive activities, and implementation of prescribed therapy.

In most cases, to intervene effectively, nurses must include both the problem and the probable etiology in the diagnostic statement. For example, consider the following three cases in which the problem of impaired skin integrity is diagnosed:

- An elderly, malnourished woman is admitted with a right-sided cerebrovascular accident. Two days later, she develops evidence of a beginning sacral decubitus.
- A 6-year-old child is seen by the school nurse for treatment of a mild knee laceration after a playground fall.
- A 35-year-old diabetic patient is referred to the community health nurse for incisional wound care management after a cholecystectomy.

Specific treatment will depend on the etiology. While the first two patients can be managed independently by the nurse, the third patient's wound care is likely to be determined in consultation with the physician.

Nursing diagnoses made on admission are based on data collected in the nursing assessment. Subsequently, these diagnoses may be validated or changed, or new ones identified, as additional data are collected. Nursing diagnoses that remain unresolved at the time of discharge must be referred for follow-up to appropriate and available resources. In most instances these will be nurses in home health agencies, in outpatient settings, or in extended care facilities.

Although still at a very early stage of development, a taxonomy for nursing diagnosis is evolving. Responsibility for coordination of professional activity in this area has been assumed by the National Conference Group for Classification of Nursing Diagnoses.* This growing, dynamic assembly of interested nurses has

---

*Address: 3525 Caroline St., St. Louis, Mo., 63104.

been actively contributing to the development of a formal taxonomy of nursing diagnoses since 1973, when Kristine Gebbie and Mary Ann Lavin called the group's first national conference at St. Louis University.[3]

The taxonomy will provide nurses with a common vocabulary to identify those patient problems for which they are accountable. The use of nursing diagnosis to more clearly define the scope of nursing practice should help to reduce the role ambiguity that has tended to evolve with the expansion of nursing practice. Nursing role clarification, in turn, will hopefully foster increased multidisciplinary collaboration and collegiality.

Standard III: *The plan of nursing care includes goals derived from the nursing diagnoses.*

Realistic goal-setting begins with assessment of the patient's goals and includes consideration of needs and resources; *patient participation in this step is mandatory*. If short- and long-term goals are identified for each problem at the time of diagnosis, discharge planning should be easier and better organized.

Nurses are responsible for defining and facilitating the achievement of patient outcomes, within a projected reasonable time frame, for the problems which they diagnose. In conjunction with the patient and members of other disciplines, the nurse designs goals that reflect the *patient's* decisions regarding the achievement and maintenance of optimum levels of health and function.

Standard IV: *The plan includes priorities and the prescribed nursing approaches or measures to achieve the goals derived from the nursing diagnoses.*

Once the nursing diagnoses and expected outcomes have been identified, plans for continued observation, prevention of complications, and therapeutic intervention can be identified. All nursing plans should be communicated clearly in the patient records, where they are available to collaborating disciplines.

Whenever resolution of a nursing diagnosis does not occur prior to discharge, plans for continued treatment should be made. Individualized plans require the participation of patient and family to create feasible, successful arrangements, particularly when referral to community agencies is involved.

Many plans can be implemented independently by the patient and significant others. For example, a diagnosis of alteration in mobility may prevent a patient in a leg cast from climbing stairs. If given enough notice, the family can adequately prepare the home environment without undue anxiety. The sooner discharge plans are solidified, the easier it will be for the family to complete arrangements.

When it becomes evident that the patient will need professional or material resources or both to meet self-care requirements after discharge, early planning again facilitates discharge. A discharge delayed because planning for home care services was postponed until the last minute is aggravating to both the patient and the staff. Even more frustrating is the decision to discharge a patient who clearly cannot manage, or be managed, at home. Arrangements for placement at extended care facilities often require days or weeks to complete. Subsequent delays, resulting in increased costs and slowed patient progress, could often be prevented with proper planning and team communication.

Standard V: *Nursing actions provide for client/patient participation in health promotion, maintenance, and restoration.*

This standard should need no explanation. If the nurse values and respects the patient's right to participate in care and corresponding decision making, efforts will be maximized to ensure that all members of the health care team provide the patient with necessary information about health status, recommendations for care, prognosis, and available resources.

The nurse must be able to articulate to the patient in clear and nonjudgmental terms the nursing diagnoses that have been made. Furthermore, discussion and demonstration of how the nurse can assist the patient to resolve these problems must also be included.

One of the most important functions of the nurse is to help the patient to delineate and evaluate options and make informed choices. The nurse then acts as the patient's advocate to see that these reasoned decisions are communicated to other health care team members so that these wishes can be carried out.

The patient's input into discharge planning should begin on the day of admission, during the initial nursing assessment, and continue throughout the course of hospitalization. To inadvertently exclude the patient would omit the nurse's most valuable source of information and might also jeopardize the patient's acceptance of a discharge plan devised in the face of limited options.

Standard VI: *Nursing actions assist the client/patient to maximize his health capabilities.*

Orem identifies five methods of assisting used by everyone at one time or another during the helping process:

1. Acting for or doing for another
2. Guiding another
3. Supporting another (physically or psychologically)
4. Providing an environment that promotes personal development in relation to becoming able to meet present or future demands for action
5. Teaching another[5,p.72]

Orem proposes that the nurse employs these approaches within the context of one of three nursing systems devised to assist the patient to achieve desired health outcomes.[5,pp.77-80] The system required by a patient helps to determine the kind of nursing help as well as the level of nursing skill required after discharge.

In a *wholly compensatory system* the patient is unable to participate in fulfilling self-care requirements; therefore the nurse primarily carries out these activities instead. The patient who remains in this system throughout the course of hospitalization usually requires either continued nursing at extended care facilities or home care nursing services. Often the patient in this category requires the help of other disciplines as well after discharge.

In the *supportive-educative system* the nurse acts primarily as a consultant, employing one or more of the last four methods of assisting to enhance the patient's self-care ability. The patient who requires such professional nursing assistance after discharge is usually referred to the visiting nurse or clinic nurse for follow-up. Referral to another discipline may also be indicated for a patient in this system.

The patient in the *partly compensatory system* works together with the nurse to meet self-care requirements; all five methods of assisting may be needed. Although this system is the one most commonly used in the acute care setting, a number of patients continue to require this type of care after discharge, in which case appropriate referral for follow-up would be anticipated.

Standard VII: *The client's/patient's progress or lack of progress toward goal achievement is determined by the client/patient and the nurse.*
Standard VIII: *The client's/patient's progress or lack of progress toward goal achievement directs reassessment, reordering of priorities, new goal setting, and revision of the plan of nursing care.*

Considered together, the final two standards direct the evaluation of discharge planning. Evaluation of nursing care is a continuous process that should be based on previously established criteria. Additionally, retrospective evaluation of nursing care can help to improve the quality of nursing care for specific populations. However, concurrent evaluation is essential if we are to recognize and correct deficiencies in goal attainment *before* the patient leaves the health care setting. Moreover, when considered within the context of discharge planning, intermittent evaluation with the patient helps to validate adequacy of the existing discharge plan or provides evidence of the need to alter the plan.

The true test comes after discharge, when the plan is implemented. In this stage the patient, as well as subsequent health care providers, can empirically validate the adequacy of discharge planning and make adjustments as indicated. If changes are required, it is essential that the independent patient be aware of appropriate health care resources that are available for consultation if needed.

A process for routine follow-up of referred patients can provide feedback about the adequacy and appropriateness of discharge planning. The continuing care consultant's liaison role can provide the link between the staff nurse and the nurse who receives the referral when direct communication between these primary providers is not possible.

DETERRENTS TO SUCCESSFUL DISCHARGE PLANNING

Several major problems interfere with the nurse's ability to participate effectively in discharge planning.

Patients in acute care settings are often seriously ill; their condition changes rapidly, but once it is stabilized, discharge may quickly follow. Hence the time available for discharge planning is shortened. Because the need for follow-up care is becoming increasingly routine, initial planning must begin on admission, with frequent reevaluation of status. In these situations careful interdisciplinary coordination and communication are mandatory and may be facilitated by routine multidisciplinary discharge planning rounds. The staff nurse directly responsible for the planning and coordination of the patient's care must see that adequate and accurate information is made available at such rounds when postdischarge care is anticipated.

Many nursing services, particularly in large medical centers, are plagued by relatively rapid staff turnovers and tightened budgets. Staffing patterns often reflect less than ideal conditions, creating situations in which crisis intervention becomes the norm and discharge planning is postponed until the day the discharge order is written.

The problem of inadequate staffing may be compounded by shift rotation and scattered days off as well as by inconsistent nursing staff assignments. Nursing care, then, may potentially be characterized by fragmentation, task orientation, and lack of continuity. In addition, nurses may not have internalized an orientation toward personal accountability for nursing practice as characterized in the ANA Standards of Nursing Practice, or they may lack the skills in nursing process required to implement the standards. The burden of responsibility for discharge planning then falls to the head nurse or continuing care consultant, neither of whom have the time to consider the comprehensive discharge needs of every patient.

PROMISING TRENDS IN PROFESSIONAL NURSING

The realities that exist in many practice settings can cause major conflicts for nurses whose values reflect the Standards of Nursing Practice. However, current developments in nursing offer hope for coping productively with these frustrations.

Trends in nursing education include a stronger focus on skill competency in the utilization of the nursing process. The incorporation of a conceptual framework for nursing practice into the curriculum enables the student to develop a clearer understanding of the roles and responsibilities of the professional nurse. Health promotion and illness prevention are being recognized to be just as much a part of nursing as health restoration. Nurses are beginning to hold themselves accountable not just for carrying out the physician's orders but for carrying out the nursing process as well. Such developments are bound to impact on nursing practice at the leadership and decision-making levels and will hopefully influence priority setting and utilization of nursing resources.

One of the most promising developments in nursing practice is primary nursing. This mode of practice places overall responsibility for the nursing care of patients in a specific case load on the individual nurse. When implemented effectively, primary nursing enables the staff nurse to plan and coordinate the patient's discharge more easily and efficiently. At the same time, primary nursing has the potential not only to improve job satisfaction but also to contribute to the professional growth of the nurse as an autonomous yet collaborative health care team member.

Primary nursing is certainly not a panacea for all the factors that interfere with effective discharge planning in nursing. However, it is this kind of professional orientation toward individual responsibility for nursing practice that will facilitate implementation of the Standards of Nursing Practice. This should benefit not only nursing but also the consumer, who has a right to expect no less.

SUMMARY

The role of the staff nurse in discharge planning involves both independent and collaborative functions. As a member of a professional discipline, the nurse diagnoses and treats distinct nursing problems, referring those which are unresolved at discharge to appropriate colleagues for continued intervention. Because of the nurse's holistic focus and continuous presence with the patient, this person is in an ideal position to facilitate the coordination and communication of discharge plans within the health care team. Nursing's specific responsibilities for discharge planning can be implemented within the framework of the American Nurses' Association Standards of Nursing Practice, which reflect the problem-solving steps of the nursing process.

REFERENCES

1. American Nurses' Association: Standards of nursing practice, Kansas City, Mo., 1973, The Association.
2. Bullough, B.: The law and the expanding nursing role, Am. J. Public Health **66**:249-254, 1976.
3. Gebbie, K. M., and Lavin, M. A.: Classifying nursing diagnoses, Am. J. Nurs. **74**:250-253, 1974.
4. Gordon, M.: Nursing diagnoses and the diagnostic process, Am. J. Nurs. **76**:1298-1300, 1976.
5. Orem, D. E.: Nursing: Concepts of Practice, New York, 1971, McGraw-Hill Book Co.
6. Soares, C.: Nursing and medical diagnoses: a comparison of variant and essential features. In Chaska, N. L., editor: The nursing profession: views through the mist, New York, 1978, McGraw-Hill Book Co.
7. Sward, K. M.: Some perspectives on ANA and quality assurance. In Issues in evaluation Research, Kansas City, Mo., 1976, American Nurses' Association.

CHAPTER 9

Discharge planning: a social worker's perspective

GUITELLE H. SANDMAN

"I want to die in my own way." "I want to die at home." "I don't want my family to watch me suffer." "Please let me stay in the hospital until I can get a little better—a little stronger." "I can't put my mother in a nursing home. It would kill her." "Who will help me when I'm home in bed?" "I know I can't take care of my baby, but I can't give him up either. What can I do?" "Who will teach me how to be a mother?" "Now that I can't work, how can I support my family? How do we eat, much less pay our medical bills?"

These quotations illustrate some of the issues that confront a social worker who is planning, with a patient, discharge from the hospital. Even when patients *want* to go home, the moment of leaving becomes frightening when they begin to realize that they will soon be assuming their former responsibilities and having to make decisions. Because these issues are of overriding importance, discharge planning has to start on or before the day of admission. The patient's life went on before entering the hospital, continued while in the hospital, and continues to go on, albeit in a changed way, after hospitalization.

In a discussion of discharge planning from a social worker's perspective, it is important to describe in a general way what social workers in a medical setting do, the theoretical framework within which they operate, and the way they function on multidisciplinary discharge planning teams. An explanation of the social worker's role as it interfaces with other disciplines in the discharge planning process will be explored. The problem-solving model of assessment, diagnosis, prescription, implementation, and evaluation will be used. Although most of the discussion of this chapter will be focused on discharge from a general hosptial, it should be noted that social work is a generic profession. Therefore the same basic principles would apply whether the patient is being discharged from an acute hospital, a chronic hospital, or a nursing home.

THEORETICAL FRAMEWORK OF SOCIAL WORK

A social worker should serve on all multidisciplinary teams. Because social workers traditionally are involved with psychosocial and relationship issues, they take care of nonmedical aspects of patient care. They have a holistic approach to the patient and family; they understand ethnic and economic issues; they know about community resources and systems; they understand ego defenses and their role in people's behavior; they can elicit background information in a nonthreatening way; they offer support. Although it is true that social workers are not unique in having these skills, the combination of the skills in a unique framework enables social workers to assist patients "who do not command the means to human subsistence in acquiring them and in attaining the highest possible degree of independence."[1] In addition, social workers have an understanding of family and group dynamics that is useful in promoting communication with both patients and staff.

Because utilization review committees mandate early discharge from hospitals, patients are frequently discharged before they are fully or independently functional. Therefore the social worker is needed to add the psychosocial dimension to the medical and nursing discharge plans. The worker assumes two roles on the team: one of direct service to the patient and the other as a consultant to the staff.

Social worker: provider of direct service

When the social worker is working directly with patients and families in a health-care setting, the following principles are employed. First, the worker tries to obtain an overview of the patient's total situation and assists in developing a conscious awareness of problems. Then the worker encourages the patient and family to communicate openly with one another and with other team members. The patient and family usually need help in adjusting emotionally to the limitations imposed by a devasting illness or to changes in their lives. They will need help in making adaptations. Therefore the social worker tries to enable the patient and family to mobilize existing problem-solving techniques and to develop new ones.

After the patient's discharge the social worker acts as a patient advocate and tries "to strengthen both formal and informal support systems at home."[2] It is not prudent to send a patient home if there is no one to provide needed care or if there are family problems with a spouse or children or another sick person. Furthermore, family "burnout," which occurs when family members become so emotionally and physically exhausted that they have nothing more to give, must also be considered. It then becomes extremely important to offer emotional support and concrete services such as financial aid, a homemaker, a visiting nurse, or transportation if the patient is mobile. In many cities there are community-based self-help and support groups that can be very useful to both patients and their families.

If a patient cannot go home, it is important to discuss alternatives with the patient and family (if the patient is attentive) or with the family members alone (if the patient is not attentive). They need to understand the reasons that make the discharge imperative and then to have as much *control* over the choices as possible. Usually many guilt feelings are aroused in family members around the time of discharge—especially if a patient is terminally ill or cannot go home. In fact, a patient may feed the guilt feelings by accusing the family of abandonment or by "acting out." That is, for no apparent organic reason the patient may suddenly become nauseous or dizzy just as the discharge plan is being discussed. This response needs to be interpreted to the family. Dealing with all these feelings then becomes a major task of the social worker. Once the plan for discharge is made, whether the patient will be transfered to another facility or will return home, the patient and family must be reassured that the staff will make every effort to facilitate the move so that the family's burden will be shared and thereby lightened.

Social worker: consultant on discharge planning team

When the social worker serves as a consultant on a multidisciplinary discharge planning team, several additional principles are involved. First, the social worker tries to point out the interpersonal dynamics within the family and with the patient. Then the worker helps the health care team to understand the significance of family, social, economic, and emotional factors that will either aid or interfere with the discharge plans. In addition, the social worker acts as an educator by providing an interpretive link between the patient and the physician, between the patient and the discharge planning team, and between the patient and the community.

Needless to say, it is also critically important to facilitate communication among the multidisciplinary team members. To do so the social worker needs to form good working relationships with the doctors and nurses, especially the latter, since it is they who are usually the source of referrals and the coordinators of discharge plans. Therefore, during meetings the social worker makes observations of problems and verbally augments notes in the medical record with pertinent information about how the patient feels about going home or who will be home to take care of the patient. Then the social worker's assessment is compared with the nurse's and is shared. After the meeting the social worker again meets with the patient to devise a reasonable, manageable plan for leaving the hospital or nursing home.

Crisis intervention

When a patient is admitted to a health care facility, the social worker needs to have an understanding of the crisis that brought the patient to the hospital and of the techniques of intervention that can be used to promote a healthy resolution of that crisis. "A crisis occurs when an individual is faced with a serious problem that seems to have no immediate solution."[3] The person then becomes abnormally anxious and upset, and regresses. Normal activities and social functions are disrupted, and the usual problem-solving mechanisms do not work. The person who has become vulnerable and frightened is more receptive to professional intervention.

If the social worker can help the person to identify the specific nature of the crisis and what caused it, the worker can then use the heightened anxiety and expression of feelings to help find solutions. In crisis intervention it is important to isolate the person's strengths and then to mobilize them in working on the crisis.[3]

For example, if a man learns that he has a malignant tumor, or if a young woman finds that she will have to lose her leg, there is a crisis. If an elderly man can no longer take care of himself alone, or if a woman has an unwanted pregnancy, a crisis is also precipitated. Since a person tends to be more responsive to someone who offers help during a crisis, the social worker can develop a relationship, establish trust, support strengths, validate feelings, and, most important, work with the patient to set priorities and find workable solutions.

DISCHARGE PLANNING PROCESS

As in all other disciplines, the social worker who is involved in discharge planning works through five steps: assessment, diagnosis, prescription, implementation, and evaluation. There must be a continuum of care that begins when the patient first comes to the clinic or hospital, progresses while he is receiving treatment in the hospital or nursing home, and extends into the home or another institution. The social worker needs to become involved with the patient and family early in the discharge process so that they will realize that the worker knows them well and cares enough about them to be their ally and advocate.

Assessment

The process of discharge planning begins when the social worker first meets the patient and begins to make an assessment that will include at least an informal psychosocial assessment of the patient's situation. After a history is taken, the worker must ascertain the patient's personality style as well as the family and ethnic backgrounds, which affect the reaction to illness. To better predict how the patient will react to the present crisis or loss, the social worker must gain an understanding of how the patient coped with crisis or loss in the past, his interests, and fears, and the family constellation. In addition, the worker tries to help the patient look realistically at himself and his situation by talking together and role playing. The worker tries to discover the patient's defenses to determine whether he will be comfortable and adaptable to changes in life-style or will be resistant and noncompliant. Once the patient's personality style is understood, the worker can more effectively work with him to find acceptable ways of dealing with the problem. Then the patient will have some sense of participation and control.

All patients have fears and anxieties about leaving the hospital and reentering the "real world"; the transition is usually difficult, even with minor illness. One patient with a chronic illness remarked that she could usually "psyche" herself into going to the hospital, but she always dreaded going home. Therefore, when a patient leaves the hospital in a more debilitated and dependent condition, financially drained, or as a new parent, the situation will assuredly be different, and the patient will probably need support or concrete help to manage the transition with some equanimity.

In considering the psychosocial needs of a patient, the social worker is alert to the patient's reactions to illness and hospitalization. The worker makes notes of the patient's procrastination in seeking help; his anxiety while waiting for results of tests or procedures; his denial, anger, resentment, hopes, and fears; the family's reactions; and finally the financial issues. The social worker must be aware of the cost of diagnosis and treatment and of managing the home while the patient is ill or recuperating. Frequently there is a prolonged loss of income, which creates a tremendous drain on family resources. Futhermore, the worker must also understand the major factors involved in rehabilitation, both physical and psychological. The social worker, with knowledge of community and health resources, as well as of hospital and governmental systems, can help the patient to work through the maze of those systems and to make appropriate use of community resources.

The social worker must be alert to specific indications of potential problems involving such chronically ill patients as (1) the functionally elderly, (2) the debilitated, (3) the excessively anxious or depressed, (4) those who can neither identify nor articulate their needs, (5) those whose physical condition changed drastically from admission to discharge (e.g., as a result of losing a body part or function), (6) those whose family situation has changed (e.g., the husband has left home, a daughter has died unexpectedly, or a son is in trouble with the law), or (7) those who might not be able to return home because of either their own illness or family problems.

In a special hospital there may be special problems. For example, in a maternity hospital there may be (1) potential problems in mothering because the patient is a teenager, did not enjoy the pregnancy, believes that the baby in utero is willfully kicking her or being "bad," does not look forward to having the baby, or has had little or poor mothering herself; (2) extraordinary medical problems, such as a cardiac or diabetic condition that would make the patient very anxious; (3) a question of adoption or abortion; (4) marital or parent-child conflicts; (5) a history of psychiatric problems; (6) indications of potential abusing patterns, such as the patient's having been a battered child herself. When these signals can be identified early in a pregnancy, more reaching out can be done, community resources can be rallied, and supports can be given and maintained.

Diagnosis

The social work diagnosis is based on the particular psychodynamic and socioeconomic factors that influenced the patient prior to illness. These factors, in turn, affect the way the patient reacts to and deals with problems connected to the present illness.

For example, if a cancer or postsurgical patient is elderly or lives alone, it behooves the social worker to look for supports from the extended family and friends and to help the patient explore personal resources.

Patient study. A 68-year-old childless widow who lived alone had a partial pelvic exenteration and then entered a rehabilitation center. After her discharge from the rehabilitation hospital, she regressed and did not care for herself. Consequently she had to be readmitted to the hospital, where she was nourished and supported. She grew to like the hospital and was reluctant to leave. The social work diagnosis of her situation was that she was phobic, partly because she had been an overprotected, only child. Also, at least in the sense that she made things difficult for herself, she seemed masochistic. Now she was pushing away the very people who wanted to help her. In assessing her personality style, the social worker saw that she dealt with losses by withdrawing from supports and was bitter, dependent, and isolated. The worker could then predict that the patient would have trouble adjusting to her colostomy and ileal conduit and would probably revert to helplessness. Therefore the worker tried to build in supports, not only for her benefit, but also for the benefit of the professionals in the community, who were frustrated by her resistance and her "help-rejecting style."

Prescription

After making the diagnosis, the social worker would make a prescription by suggesting ways of helping the patient and family cope with altered mobility or function with a changed family situation. For example, on a visiting nurse referral the social worker would delineate potential problems from a psychosocial point of view. It might be suggested that because a patient has trouble adjusting to even minor changes, the care givers should have the patience to frequently repeat their instructions and the reasons change is needed. A patient who has trouble being independent may need creative encouragement in self-care. A patient who "enjoys" illness may need to discuss this tendency with someone who will help him overcome it and find ways to have self-satisfactions that are less costly. For example, the social worker might try to find some meaningful people in the patient's life and then help him focus at least part of his time on others rather than on himself.

A common problem in designing a specific discharge plan involves the lack of available community resources. Many persons need extra household help when they go home and expect to obtain it without paying. The social worker might agree that they need help but knows that there is no third-party payment for most people. Thus the worker explores with the patient and family members what *they* see as resources. Whom could they call for help? Where could they obtain money to pay for it? Could they possibly manage without help by changing their expectations of themselves until the patient is stronger? In exploring these quesitons the patient and worker together can frequently find creative alternatives to compensate for the lack of community resources.

Many patients who are about to leave the hospital expect to have the services of a visiting nurse or at least a homemaker to help until they are more self-sufficient. Unfortunately these expectations are unrealistic, since the visiting nurse must limit her time to meeting skilled nursing needs. Futhermore, the fees charged by homemakers are high. Therefore, although the social worker might ideally prescribe the services of a homemaker, in the discharge plan, realistically it might not be feasible to obtain such services.

Similar problems occur when a patient needs to enter a nursing home. If the level of nursing care required is skilled, there is little difficulty unless there is a shortage of "skilled beds." If, however, only minimum nursing care is needed, even though the patient might be terminally ill and bedridden, there is usually no third-party coverage (Medicaid legislation sometimes allows an exception). It is understandable that when patients realize these services are not available, they and their families become angry, and much of that anger at the "system" is directed toward the social worker. Consequently the more problems can be anticipated, and the better communication there is among team members in terms of delineating and documenting patient needs, the less frustrating and the more successful a discharge plan is likely to be.

Implementation

Implementation primarily consists of documenting the patient's discharge problems and carrying out specific follow-up details. For example, immediately after discharge, the social worker makes telephone calls to determine how the patient is doing and whether the patient is inordinately depressed, the visiting nurse is coming, or Meals on Wheels has arrived. If the worker and patient already have a good relationship, communication is likely to be more candid and the assessment of the patient's situation more accurate.

Evaluation

There are some problems in evaluating the social worker's part of the discharge plan. Unless home visits (which are not cost-effective on a regular basis) or extended telephone calls are made, it is difficult to know how the plan has worked. Therefore it is advantageous to have some mechanism for evaluation within the program, such as simple follow-up forms that can be filled out by the visiting nurse, nursing home, or community agency and thus can provide some feedback on the efficacy of the discharge plan. The evaluation forms would usually be returned to the coordinator of the discharge planning team but could be sent to any represented discipline having responsibility in an area in which a problem has arisen.

When a patient has been transferred to another facility such as a nursing home, the social worker should make at least one visit either alone or with another team member. To both the patient and the nursing home these visits indicate that the discharge planning team is interested in the patient's *continuing care* and that, in fact, the patient has been neither abandoned nor "dumped." On occasion, if the placement has not been satisfactory, work to change the plan can be started. No plan has to be permanent; in fact, it should be flexible enough to present more than one option.

CASE STUDIES FROM A SOCIAL WORK PERSPECTIVE

The best way to show how multidisciplinary teams actually work and how the social worker functions on the team would be to describe a few cases that illustrate some of the issues that arise.

Case 1. Mrs. J., 52 years of age, was known to our clinic for many years because she was a "cured" cancer patient left with a draining fistula and osteoporosis. She always presented herself in a whining, complaining manner, so that she tended to alienate those who wanted to help her. She was widowed and had nine children, none of whom still lived at home. Her medical problems were extensive: she had a drinking problem, she had terrible odor from her fistula, and she was crippled. The staff felt that she was also manipulative. She either would not keep her clinic appointments or would come at the wrong time; she regulated her own medication; and she refused offers of homemaking help but then complained because she could not manage alone.

As a result of her personality style, Mrs. J. did not receive the kind of care she needed, and all the workers involved were frustrated. Appointments were made for her for various consultations, but she frequently did not keep them.

It became clear at a multidisciplinary team meeting that all members had to change the way they dealt with Mrs. J. They examined what was happening and tried to analyze why everyone was feeling so upset and "used." It appeared that limits had to be set not only for Mrs. J. but also for what staff members could expect from themselves. The visiting nurse was particularly frustrated because she felt sabotaged by Mrs. J., and yet felt that the ultimate responsibilty for Mrs. J.'s care rested on her. The team supported the nurse by affirming that she was not alone and that everyone understood her problems and admired her perseverance. Futhermore, no one expected miracles from her.

In turn, Mrs. J. had to know that she had some choices. She could follow through with plans made with her through the clinic, or she could go to another facility. If she chose the latter, she could receive help in making the transition but then would have to be responsible for going to the new hospital and for following through on her care. Homemaking and friendly visitor help could be obtained for her, but she would have to be responsible for being home at designated times or for informing workers of a change in plans. She had to know that if she did not keep her part of the bargain, the services would have to be withdrawn. She would have to be honest with physicians, nurses, and social workers; she could not continue to relate one set of symptoms to one physician and change those symptoms for another. Her rights and our limits were pointed out and seemed acceptable to her. Because she has multiple needs, she will always need help in dealing with the medical system. She had to learn that acceptable ways of asking for help will be successful and that unacceptable methods are likely to be unsuccessful.

The staff members also had to learn to talk to one another, to corroborate their observations, and to make a concerted plan that was feasible to implement. They had to share their frustrations, explore why they were so angry, and support each other. In fact, Mrs. J. chose to go to a neighborhood health clinic, where she seems to be satisfied with her care. This case indicated that it is better to set firm limits, to give clear options for the patient's control, and then to facilitate a transfer.

In another complicated case there was more involvement with the family than with the patient.

Case 2. Mrs. S., 63 years of age, was seen on her first clinic appointment, which she had put off for seven months as she watched her symptoms become more severe.

At the clinic she was told that she had a large abdominal mass, that she would have to be hospitalized, and that her condition was serious. The social worker was called because her 26-year-old daughter was extremely upset. The daughter, Kathy, had known that Mrs. S. was sick but had been unable to persuade her to have an examination. The worker spoke with Kathy and tried to help her understand that she should not blame herself for her mother's obstinacy. Mrs. S., meanwhile, was rather stoical and in many ways was relieved to be in the hospital. Thus the first contact with family was in a time of crisis, when both patient and daughter were responsive to social work intervention.

Mrs. S. came from a large, extended Italian family. Her husband was a retired fisherman who was on disability because of cataracts and poor eyesight. The patient had two children—a married son, 28 years of age, who was not eager to become involved, and Kathy, who was divorced and lived with her parents and her 6-year-old son, Richie.

While the patient was hospitalized for surgery, she was discussed weekly at multidisciplinary meetings. The team discussed not only the patient's actual physical condition but also her feeling about what was happening and the family's reaction to her situation. Plans for discharge began early. The social worker's diagnosis was that Kathy was assuming too much of the burden and would need help in setting realistic limits for herself.

During Mrs. S.'s hospitalization the thrust of social work efforts was directed toward Kathy, since other family members were only tangentially involved. Frequently Kathy would spend an hour with the social worker before visiting with her mother, or she would come down afterward to cry or to talk over what was going on at home. The social worker and Kathy discussed Richie and what to tell him about his grandmother's illness. They also discussed his nightmares and anxiety, trying to work out comfortable ways to help him deal with his sadness and fears.

As Mrs. S. reached the point where discharge was imminent, there were frequent team meetings, which usually included the family and the visiting nurse. At these meetings everyone talked about Mrs. S.'s desire to die at home, about the family's financial distress (Mrs. S. had neither insurance nor Medicaid), about the need for special equipment in the home, and about the patient's particular medical needs, prognosis, and personality. (Mrs. S. had become quite demanding.) Kathy was given guidelines, and was taught how to set limits and to ask for help. She was also urged to give some time to herself so that she would not "burn out."

When the patient was discharged, she had to come to the clinic regularly so that her condition could be monitored, and she wanted Kathy to accompany her. Therefore Kathy was encouraged to come alone for an extra hour each week so that she could cry, ventilate, be angry, or just talk about her own feelings and needs. She learned that she could call any member of the team if a problem arose, no matter what the hour. In fact, she did so when necessary.

At multidisciplinary team meetings after discharge, the visiting nurse joined the team. She gave her perceptions not only of the patient's medical condition but also of the family's coping style. Together the team worked on ways to help Mrs. S. feel more productive and in control. Because Mrs. S. wanted to see Richie read and to see Kathy remarry, she had an incentive to participate in her care. When she had something to look forward to, she could deal better emotionally with her progressive disfigurement and dependence.

When it became clear that Mrs. S.'s condition was terminal, "the door was left open" for Kathy to call if she felt she could not handle the situation any longer at home. It was Mrs. S., however, who indicated when she needed to come back to the hospital, and in fact she died a few days after her final admission.

The social worker's relationship with Kathy, and tangentially with the S. family, lasted a year. Kathy continued to come every other week and used this treatment appropriately as she discussed her problems and worked on her grief. Kathy felt that she had grown from the experience, and although she was sad, she felt that there were many positive aspects. Mainly she felt that people cared about her.

In this case the initial assessment indicated that Mrs. S. was to have a colostomy and would leave the hospital in a dependent role, which would be difficult for her. It was noted that she was a feisty woman who liked to be in control. She also enjoyed her nourishing role. From her history it was learned that she had a large, extended Italian family in which it was permissible for people to show their emotions; that is, they could cry or be angry and still be supported. It was learned also that Mrs. S. was "the strong one" in the family and that she had set a model for Kathy to follow in terms of caring for sick parents.

The social work diagnosis was that there would be problems after discharge in persuading Mrs. S. and Kathy to accept the help they needed; there also would be problems in persuading them to apply for the finanical assistance they needed.

Clearly the social work prescription concurred with that of medical and nursing staff. Kathy and Mrs. S. needed considerable instruction and support to accept the help they needed. A visiting nurse came twice daily. Hill-Burton funds were obtained for Mrs. S., as well as disability payments. Implementation of the plan was carried out by the visiting nurse, by follow-up clinic visits, by obtaining medicabs and ambulances when needed, and by keeping channels of communication open, especially for Kathy. Evaluation took place during multidisciplinary follow-up meetings and was facilitated by the social worker's long involvement with Kathy and her willingness to participate.

A final case shows how being alert to potential problems with a maternity patient helps in making an intial assessment and diagnosis early so that the prescription for prolonged care can be carefully designed and implemented.

Case 3. Mrs. D., 30 years of age, presented to the medical prenatal clinic when she was five months pregnant. She was the eleventh of twelve children; both parents were alcoholics; she had been beaten as a child; her home was very disorganized. She herself had not had good mothering. This pregnancy was the outcome of a short-lived affair, but because she had wanted a child, she was pleased, at first, to be pregnant. The social worker had considerable involvement with her during that time because the pregnancy was complicated by a severe congenital heart problem. Because, during the pregnancy, Mrs. D. focused much more on herself than on the baby, the staff members were alert to problems. In fact, once her little boy was born, she had a temporary psychotic episode and did not want to care for her child. The worker was very concerned about Mrs. D.'s ability to create a bond with the baby.

During the pregnancy there were frequent multidisciplinary meetings in the clinic to reality-test, since Mrs. D. was skillful at pitting one professional against another and distorting information that was given to her. She had no interest in the new baby but was more concerned with her own survival. She felt that the baby was deliberately trying to hurt her.

During the pregnancy doctors and nurses patiently and repeatedly explained what was happening to Mrs. D. and the need for the various medications, tests, procedures, and hospital admission. A community health nurse was contacted to monitor her condition at home and also to build a relationship so that follow-up could continue postnatally. Since this patient was particularly manipulative, multidisciplinary team meetings were useful to everyone involved, including doctors, ambulatory care nurses, community health nurses, and social workers. The team members could listen to each other, feel less alone and frustrated, and *gain support from each other,* which was an invaluable adjunct. Since so much attention was given to the patient prenatally, she began to trust "helping people," which was very difficult for her, and to accept the discharge plans. After much deliberation, she kept her baby. However she will continue to need considerable support from all disciplines, as well as from many community agencies, such as the VNA, the welfare department, and day care facilities. Even though she and the baby are doing well, the social worker still sees her to give emotional support, acts as liaison between her and the agencies supplying the ongoing services she requires, and also offers support to the community agencies.

SOCIAL WORKER AS MULTIDISCIPLINARY TEAM MEMBER

Most persons who enter the social work profession do so because they like people and want to help make their lives better. They like to be involved by helping to improve coping skills and by making whatever environmental changes are feasible. Therefore, when they are able to work for a long period of time with a patient on a discharge plan, they receive considerable satisfaction. The social workers become closely connected to the patient and family and can understand how they functioned and coped. They can also observe and implement changes within the family system. Although it is more gratifying to work with patients over a long period of time, it is also rewarding to do short-term work. There is a challenge and stimulation in having to do a quick, thorough assessment for a discharge plan. When those plans involve other disciplines, as they usually do, there is satisfaction in seeing "the parts of a puzzle fit together" and a viable plan come forth. Nevertheless, when a patient leaves the hospital, the staff members need to understand their own feelings of loss as they say good-bye. If there is a good mechanism for obtaining feed-back on how the patient is doing and how the discharge plan has worked, staff members will have greater satisfaction. A good discharge plan means not only that concrete and health care needs are met but also that communication and understanding have been facilitated.

Myths to be confronted

There are many social work myths that are frustrating to the worker and should be dispelled. For example, social workers themselves tend to have rescue fantasies and would like to make everything all right for their patients. Instead, they must realize that just as doctors, nurses, and therapists of all kinds cannot cure everyone, neither can social workers necessarily change the life or personality style of every patient nor improve every social or economic situation. They can only try to make improvements where possible. They need to accept their own limitations as well their patients', and to help other disciplines do the same.

Another problem for all workers in a health care setting lies in dealing with some of the harsh realities and misperceptions that people have. For example, many patients believe that if they have medical insurance, they will have no medical expenses. Obviously, for those who have incomplete coverage, the expenses can become overwhelming. Many expenses, such as for household help, are simply not covered by third-party payments. Other patients believe that since they have given to organizations such as the American Cancer Society (ACS), they will then reap the benefits of these donations when they become sick. They expect unlimited transportation, equipment, and even money from ACS, but there are restrictions on the use of available funds.

Another problem often heard is that patients should be able to stay in the hospital until they are well or at least until they are strong enough to care for themselves. They have little understanding of the purpose of utilization review committees. The social worker is then faced with early discharge for resistant patients or families and with the need to help people to obtain transitional services (e.g., transportation, housing, and household help) that are not readily available.

SUMMARY

In summary, the social worker's role on a multidisciplinary team for discharge planning is to explain and manage the psychosocial elements of patient care. The social worker carries out this assignment both directly and as a consultant. Patient needs and social situations have to be assessed early to ascertain what supports are available and what will be needed. The social worker needs to understand the patient's fears of being "different," of dying, or of being abandoned or alone. The worker needs to recognize that the family fears watching a loved one die, deteriorate, or enter a nursing home. Families need help in dealing with their own limitations of time and energy. Once a clear assessment of the situation has been made, the social worker makes a diagnosis and prescribes a social work plan to be implemented at home or in another facility. Then there is a need for both the social worker and family to be satisfied with the plan and to be able to evaluate how it has worked. Therefore the social work role in the discharge planning process is to understand the effects of illness on the patient and family and then with the patient's participation and in conjunction with other disciplines, work toward supportive, cooperative discharge planning.

REFERENCES

1. Crouch, R. C.: Social work defined, Social Work **24**:46-49, 1979.
2. Sacolick, L.: How we communicate: a case presentation to a hospital auxiliary board, Social Work in Health Care **2**:311-317, 1977.
3. Smith, L. L.: Crisis intervention in practice, Social Casework **60**:81-88, 1979.

ADDITIONAL READINGS

Caputi, M. A.: Social Work in health care: past and future, Health Soc. Work **3**:8-27, 1978.

Rapoport, L.: The state of crisis; some theoretical considerations. In Parad, H. J., editor: Crisis intervention: selected readings, New York, 1974, Family Service Association of America, pp. 22-31.

Selected papers from the March and October, 1969, Institutes for Physicians, Nurses, Social Workers, and Related Personnel Concerned With the Continuity of Health Care, held at the Training and Information Center for Home Health and Related Community Services, Montefiore Hospital Association of Western Pennsylvania, in Pittsburgh:

Calvert, M. F.: Stimulating interest and response in post-hospital care, Pittsburgh, 1970, pp. 55-61.

Coleman, M.: Community health needs and the implications for education, Pittsburgh, 1970, pp. 179-189.

Cooper, E.: Guidelines for discharge planning from the point of view of the social worker, Pittsburgh, 1970, pp. 117-127.

Mitchell, J.: Stimulating community interest and response in post-hospital care, Pittsburgh, 1970, pp. 39-45.

CHAPTER 10

Discharge planning: a physician's perspective

ROBERT J. MASTER

For elderly, chronically ill, and medically complex patients the most glaring care deficiency encountered is the virtual absence of approaches that provide continuity of care in an individualized and accountable way. For these populations, often the most important decisions relate to resource allocation, technology use, and placement options. These decisions, which are necessary to promote function, comfort, and emotional support, have little in common with "acute" medical care but nonetheless are usually made by the acute care hospital simply because no one else can do so. Although there should be an abundance of accessible, well-organized, community-based primary care systems for these populations, there are none. Whereas the hospital should be involved only in those acute situations that require a high level of technologic and personnel resources, it is in reality involved in many more.

A variety of factors produce and perpetuate this inappropriate and expensive reliance on the hospital. Some of these factors include the clear emergence of the hospital as the centralized resource of medical technology,[14] the narrow scope and isolated patterns of traditional physician practice, and the underdeveloped use of nonphysician primary care practitioners. In addition there is an array of regulatory and reimbursement policies that inhibit the development of primary care efforts appropriately focused on those persons most in need of an alternative to the hospital. It is in the cities where the care delivery environment is so skewed by the large teaching hospitals that the impact of all these factors is most pronounced; paradoxically, as will be described, it is also where experimental alternatives have had the greatest opportunity to develop.

URBAN HEALTH CARE: ROLE OF THE URBAN HOSPITAL

In urban settings it is clear that the population whose impact is greatest on hospitals is the one for which primary care systems are most underdeveloped. Middle-income, white collar, professional, relatively healthy individuals have been the marketing target of the health maintenance organization. The less affluent, pediatric, young adult, and obstetrical populations have been the target of neighborhood health centers. For the urban elderly, medically fragile, and chronically ill homebound and nursing home populations, primary care efforts have been isolated and incomplete, with the following consequences: the very people who most need a thoughtful, individualized approach to care and technology utilization are the ones who rarely have an option other than the large teaching hospital.

The elderly in particular represent those persons who are at greatest risk for hospital contact. The over-65 age group is by far the least healthy segment of the population. One fourth lives alone, and 20% have incomes below the poverty level. Surveys indicate a significant prevalence of chronic illness and disability. Individuals over 65 years of age average 36.5 days of restricted activity and 14.1 days of bed disability per year. Eighty percent have one or more chronic condition, 17.6% have mobility limitations, 5.2% are completely homebound, and 5% require a nursing home.[3,4]

The plight of the elderly and homebound in the inner city is particularly tragic. Physical disability is compounded by extreme economic hardship, social isolation, and a virtual absence of easily accessible physicians.[1,2,5] For illness there is usually no alternative but the emergency room. All too often the encounter leads to hospitalization and an exlusive focus on pathophysiologic events, acute illness, and technologic intervention.

Once the patient enters the hospital, two common scenarios are played out. In the first the patient is ultimately returned home, often with complex care plans and inadequate primary care follow-up and with a high risk of readmission as a consequence of unmonitored deterioration. The second scenario is placement in a chronic disease hospital or a nursing home after a determination that community-based resources are simply inadequate to support a return home.

NURSING-HOME PATIENTS: A SPECIAL NEED

Many studies have documented the high prevalence of disease and disability among nursing-home patients as well as the widespread difficulties they encounter in receiving adequate medical care.[7,12,13] In urban, low-income communities the number of available physicians is low, and *neighborhood health centers have had no impact on this population*.[10] In addition, current regulatory and reimbursement policies produce disincentives to the provision of medical care in the nursing-home setting.[11] Finally, it has been pointed out that physicians often avoid nursing homes because of a constellation of negative attitudes toward aging and chronic illness, an avoidance that is reinforced by the nonprofessional nature of many homes.[15]

As a consequence it is the hospital that assumes the major responsibility for the medical care of urban nursing-home patients. Ongoing care occurs in the outpatient departments, and episodic problems, from the most trivial to the life threatening, are handled in the emergency units. There is little if any continuity of care.

In essence, the only option for the elderly and chronically ill populations, which are most in need of individualized care, is to receive care as a by-product of active training programs. These programs are organized with a disease and specialty orientation, often more for the convenience of those providing the service than of those receiving it, and as a consequence the care givers are unable to understand or deal with the complex needs of these populations.

Because physicians determine who will be hospitalized and what the content of that hospitalization will be, the admitting physician (often a house officer in urban teaching hospitals) can ameliorate the consequences of this discontinuity by some basic actions. First, at the time of admission it is crucial for the physician to look beyond the issues that narrowly relate to acute illness. Relevant questions should include some of the following: Where did this patient come from, and is a return to the same place possible? If so, what additional supports will be required? If not, what is an appropriate alternative?

The purpose of these questions is *not* to impose one's judgment or values where there is little experience or training but rather to start the process in which the patient, family, and others in the hospital can look at the issues early, before compromises are required by pressures to expedite discharge.

Ultimately the decision as to where one goes after hospitalization is solely that of the patient or family. The hospital-based professional who seems to be in the best position to facilitate that decision is the floor nurse caring for the patient. This is particularly true in hospitals organized around the primary nursing concept, where an identifiable nurse teams with the physician and members of other disciplines to assume parallel management responsibility for the patient.

As most hospitalizations proceed, acute medical management evolves into chronic care management, and decisions relating to function, comfort, and placement assume greater importance than decisions relating to diagnosis and therapy. As this occurs, if the physician can allow the predominant care responsibility to be assumed by the nurse, and if the nurse is allowed to function as a primary coordinator of care, mobilizing other disciplines (e.g., physical therapy, occupational therapy, social service, and discharge planning units) on behalf of the patient, the outcome of hospitalization has a better chance of being consistent with the goals of the patient or family.

In most instances it seems that physician priorities do not allow a broader perspective, and hospital nursing responsibilities are still far too restricted. Add to this restriction a complex patient with multidimensional problems who is lacking ongoing primary care, and one has the continuity vacuum so prevalent today. Into this vacuum, which exists for the most complex and fragile patients, who are least able to control their destiny, are placed the hospital discharge planning units. In most hospitals these units endeavor to mobilize multidisciplinary talents on behalf of the patient, but they are generally perceived by physicians as being a convenient placement service for patients whose acute illness has been treated but who have no place to go. In reality, members of discharge planning teams may be the only workers in the entire hospital-based care delivery process who attempt to evaluate the total care needs of the patient while attempting to put together a patchwork of facilities and services in an attempt to meet that particular patient's needs.

Clearly, however, hospital-based discharge planning programs cannot be the final answer. Discharge planning teams, although reasonably effective, are only stopgaps in a totally discontinuous, fragmented care delivery system. They are the consequence of inadequate care delivery, not the solution. However successful they may be, discharge planning efforts should be viewed only as a palliative until such time as truly comprehensive primary care systems are in place.

THE PHYSICIAN IN TRADITIONAL PATTERNS OF PRACTICE: AN INADEQUATE APPROACH TO THE COMPLEX PATIENT

Historically, physicians have approached the problems of inadequate primary care as though a care delivery vacuum existed outside their domain. To a great extent this approach reflects the imperatives of private practice and the high level of performance physicians have asked of themselves, as well as the unrealistic expectations the public has of physicians. Public expectations have also been translated into public policy. Currently, physician services are the only reimbursable primary care services in most settings, and legally, physicians often must initiate, take responsibility for, or ratify actions of all other care providers.

The effect of all these factors is to identify solutions to the problem of discontinuity solely in terms of physician activities. There is an assumption that no one else is capable of assuming primary care responsibility and that as a consequence the physician can and must be all things to all people in all settings where care is required.

However, physicians are not present in all settings. In low-income communities, physicians in a total practice pattern are rare or nonexistent.[5] In other communities, where physicians are organized in total practice modes, it is unusual to find a physician who can manage patients continuously through the ambulatory, home, extended care facility, and hospital setting. The logistics required to remain efficient in both ambulatory and hospital practice would allow only token home care and nursing-home contact.

More importantly, even if physicians did (or could) manage their high-risk patients through all these settings, the level of involvement possible would allow response only to unidimensional pathophysiologic changes. Ultimately, this aspect of care, which is the primary focus of the physician, may be the least important for most individuals in these populations.

For example, an elderly, home-bound patient with progressive dementia, congestive heart failure, and renal insufficiency is often propelled toward the hospital and the nursing home, not by issues relating to the titration of digoxin, diuretics, or major tranquilizers, but usually because of problems relating to function, family support, or the ability of family members to cope. Evaluation of these problems requires an enormous amount of time. In addition, they are generally outside the areas of physician training and interest, and they cannot be adequately handled amid the other clinical demands on the busy physician.

The view that physicians alone can impact positively on the discontinuous nature of care currently received by these high-risk populations is unfair to the public and to the physician. Myths of omniscience and omnipresence are perpetuated. Expectations are preserved that are impossible to meet. Reality is blatantly ignored.

THE ALTERNATIVE: A CONTINUUM OF PRIMARY CARE THROUGH A MULTIDISCIPLINARY APPROACH

If there is to be a meaningful alternative to the patterns of care that currently exist, it must occur through models that are universally accessible, available around the clock, indivudalized, and, above all, continuous. Such an alternative can occur only through the development of multidisciplinary primary care teams that provide individualized care, advocacy, and allocation of resources in whatever the setting, be it home, office, hospital, or extended care facility. Since no one professional can be everywhere and do everything, a team appraoch with clear diffusion of responsibility is not just desirable, *it is essential*.

The crucial challenge, then, is to define who should be that primary agent and coordinator of care in each setting, as well as how the workers in the various settings will be linked together and reimbursed. The physician is the most expensive and scarce component of the comprehensive care model. Therefore physician time should be efficiently spent in caring for patients who have acute or ongoing medically complex problems or who require hospitalization for subspecialty intervention. It is a poor (and perhaps impossible) allocation of a scarce resource to make the physician a monitor of chronic illness, coordinator of care, and determiner of support service utilization for long-term care service patients. Yet, current regulatory and reimbursement policy is based on the assumption that the physician must perform all these functions, and the results are predictable. A paper compliance occurs that bears little resemblance to reality.

Who, then, should be working as a partner with the physician as the primary agent of care, coordinator of services, and allocator of resources for the long-term care patient (homebound patient or nursing-home resident) as well as the more medically stable, ambulatory patients? This person could be a community health nurse with expanded skills, a clinical nurse specialist or other primary care clinical specialist, or a nurse practitioner.[16] In Boston innovative approaches to the care of nursing-home and homebound populations have demonstrated that the nurse practitioner is ideally suited for this role when functioning in a close working relationship with nurses, home health aides, social workers, physical therapists, and other health workers and with close physician collaboration.[6,10] For patients cared for primarily by nurse practitioners in these experimental approaches, the results were translated into a significant decrease in hospital use, excellent patient and family satisfaction, and considerable cost savings.[6,10]

In the experienced and appropriately trained nurse practitioner seem to be merged all the disciplines required to make a comprehensive medical, nursing, rehabilitative, and resource requirement evaluation as well as to provide monitoring and first-level intervention for episodic medical problems. In the experimental systems that have been operational in Boston for over five years, it has been shown that a full-time nurse practitioner can care for approximately 120 mixed skilled nursing facility (SNF) and intermediate-level nursing-home patients or 50 mixed intensive and intermediate-level homebound individuals[6,10,17] and make sufficient visits to make a living at a reimbursement rate of approximately $20 per visit.

In addition to the physician and the nurse practitioner, team support personnel should be present and accountable to the coordinator of care for each patient. These team members are most important in home care, where family support supplements are often the crucial variable in determining whether a patient can be maintained at home or whether nursing home placement will be necessary. Such support personnel include, as a minimum, neighborhood-based homemaker/home health aides, social workers, and physical therapists. Experience in Boston with homemaker/home health aides has demonstrated that if they are selected from the neighborhood in which they work and are trained by, and accountable to, nurses who continue to work with them, the problems of performance, morale, and turnover often found in agency personnel can be reduced.[8] Currently the only mechanism for reimbursement of these support services would be placement under the aegis of a certified home care agency.

In 1977 in Boston a city-wide care delivery experiment was initiated that created or modified three certified home care programs in geographically distinct sections of the city. These programs were linked to a physician–nurse practitioner group practice that provided ambulatory care through four neighborhood health centers, nursing-home care through a contract arrangement with the Massachusetts Department of Public Welfare, and hospital care to patients in the system. An attempt was made to identify the problems that produced the discontinuous nature of care for urban high-risk populations and to develop creative organizational and reimbursement approaches to provide a "continuum of care" where previously none had existed.[9]

The system links five primary care physicians, twelve nurse practitioners, three certified home care programs employing social workers, physical therapists, and neighborhood-based homemaker/home health aides, four neighborhood health centers, an experimental nursing-home component, and a major urban hospital. Currently nearly 400 homebound and 400 nursing-home patients are cared for by the

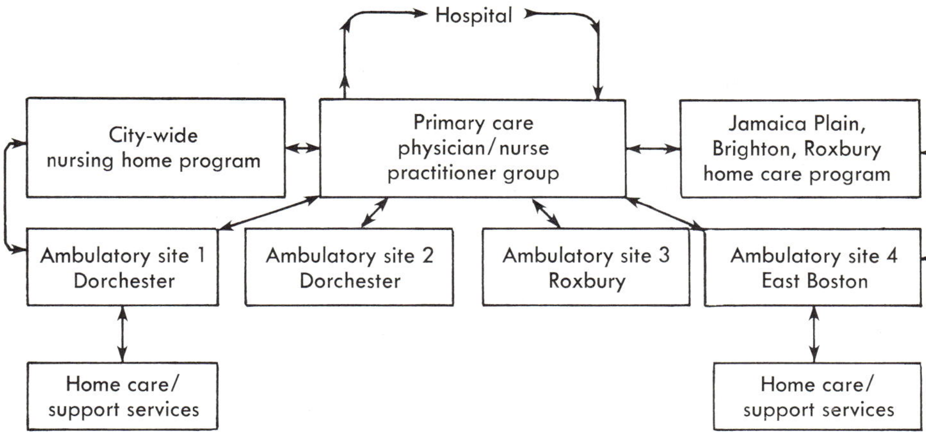

Fig. 10-1. Boston experimental health care delivery system.

system, in addition to nearly 4,000 ambulatory patients burdened with a high prevalence of chronic illness and disability (Fig. 10-1).

The nurse practitioners function as the primary agents of care for homebound patients and nursing-home residents as well as for the more stable ambulatory population. The physicians, in addition to maintaining ambulatory practices in the neighborhood health centers, provide backup for the nurse practitioners as well as maintain round-the-clock coverage for all of the population served. Most importantly, they provide continuity when hospitalization is required. The entire spectrum of support personnel is available to the nurse practitioners under the auspices of the three home care programs.

With such a system in place, and geographically distributed throughout urban communities, hospital involvement has been reduced or eliminated for a wide range of issues that have nothing to do with acute illness. Currently hospitals must function as a "central clearinghouse" for homebound individuals who require nursing-home placement, nursing-home patients who require a more sophisticated level of care, ambulatory patients who require a short-term nursing-home stay, and so on. In addition, hospitals must deal with an entire spectrum of problems that occur because no other agency exists to solve them.

With the alternative of primary care multidisciplinary teams, patients, wherever they are in the system, are medically enfranchised and can be cared for, in an individualized fashion and in whatever setting is appropriate, by a transfer of care responsibility from one member of the team to another. Movement from the home to the nursing home and back, or from ambulatory care to home care or nursing-home care, becomes an internal matter and is determined by the patient, family,

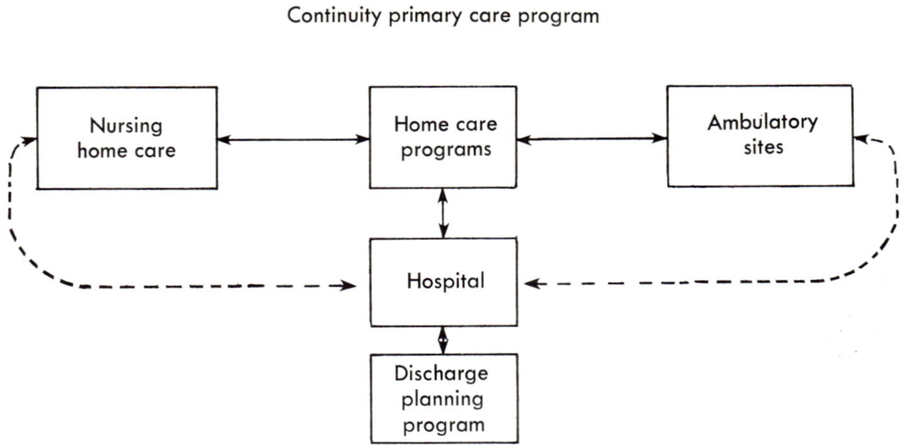

Fig. 10-2. System of primary care in which a multidisciplinary team provides continuity in the delivery of care.

and care team. The hospital becomes extraneous to this process and is used only for acute, complicated, or highly technologic health problems (Fig. 10-2).

REALITY: BARRIERS INHIBITING DEVELOPMENT OF PRIMARY CARE SYSTEMS FOR URBAN HIGH-RISK POPULATIONS

Currently a number of barriers in urban communities effectively perpetuate discontinuous care and dependence on the hospital. A primary barrier is the prevailing posture of the urban teaching hospital, which effectively perpetuates the inequities of care that have always been borne by urban low-income residents. In many centers the predominant academic attitude is that good training occurs only through full-time, hospital-based strucutres unencumbered by community physicians, and thus a mass of persons who are medically disenfranchised and lack health care options are required. In Boston and other urban centers, some teaching hospitals actively inhibit the development of primary care systems in the communities that have traditionally provided their "teaching material" by refusing to recognize the right of the urban primary care physicians to exercise control of the care of their patients in the hospital. Until the large teaching hospitals embrace the notion that physician training can no longer derive its strength from the plight of those who lack options, the problem of providing rational primary care to these high-risk populations will remain unsolvable and the concept of "continuity" an abstraction.

A second barrier is embodied in reimbursement policies that skew all the incentives to the provision of care in the hospital. With the exception of an experimental effort in Boston, no third-party payer recognizes any provider of nursing-home primary care other than the physician. In addition, reimbursement for physician services is so limited that it is financially impossible to provide substantive, ongoing care in the nursing home even if all the other disincentives to physician involvement are removed. A prerequisite for the transfer of care from the hospital to the nursing home must be a reimbursement policy that recognizes the legitimacy and necessity of ongoing care in long-term care settings. Crucial to this approach would be reimbursement for nurse practitioners or other primary care providers whose role involves total patient management and coordination of service in the context of comprehensive care programs.

Home care reimbursement policy is currently so restrictive as to make all but supplemental skilled nursing services and some limited support services impossible to deliver. Visit limits and severe restrictions as to the type of problems that will be reimbursed characterize the Medicare reimbursement policy and ignore the heterogeneous nature and needs of the homebound patient. On the one hand there is an extremely medically fragile group of homebound patients (intensive as defined by Trager[17]) whose basic limitation stems from active medical illness such as recurrent congestive heart failure, pneumonia, dehydration, infections seen as the complications of advanced cardiac disease, advanced pulmonary disease, advanced cancer, or terminal complications. In this group, predictably, there is a higher demand for medical services and a high risk for admission to a hospital. For this group, home care alternatives must include physician, nurse practitioner, nursing, and support services on a continuing basis unencumbered by restrictions on the number of visits that are reimbursable.

The other end of the homebound spectrum is characterized by persons who do not have active illness but whose limiting factor is physical disability (intermediate and basic levels, as delineated by Trager[17]). Such persons are homebound because of decreased mobility secondary to cerebrovascular accident, advanced arthritis, or severe sensory impairment, or because of various degrees of dementia that make exit from a familiar setting inordinately risky. Persons who are homebound primarily because of chronic disability rather than the consequences of active illness are most at risk for nursing-home placement. Home care efforts here must focus on support services that substitute for the family or supplement what the family is able to do, such as homemaker/home health aide service, transportation, and meal service. If nursing-home placement via the hospital is to be avoided, these services must be reimbursed without restriction, despite the fact that ongoing skilled nursing care cannot be justified.

A third barrier to the development of appropriate primary care systems is embodied in the unrealistic public expectations of physicians, which assume that only physicians can legitimately provide primary care. These expectations are sadly reinforced by regulatory policy. Currently only the physician can order home care or nursing-home services, prescribe medications, and sign death certificates. Although there are few services that are actually performed, supervised, or even known to the physician in long-term care, in theory at least, no medical ancillary, nursing, social work, or rehabilitative service can be provided to any patient unless ordered by or directly supervised by a physician. Such public expectations and regulatory policies ignore reality, demean the contribution of other care providers, and provide additional incentives toward the abdication of care responsibility to the hospital.

If alternative approaches are to be established, regulatory policy must recognize that diffusion of care delivery responsibility to nurse practitioners (or similar primary care clinicians) is desirable, necessary, and consistent with reality. Nurse practitioners should be recognized as legitimate agents of care for homebound and nursing-home patients. Nurse practitioners should be able to prescribe, under their own license, well-delineated categories of medication as well as sign death certificates. Finally, nurse practitioners should be as accountable for all activities that occur under their supervision as the physician traditionally has been.

SUMMARY

In summary, an impressive array of forces effectively inhibits the development of primary care alternatives to the discontinuous systems of care that are in place for disenfranchised, high-risk populations. Consequently those persons involved in hospital-based discharge planning efforts must continue to "keep their finger in the dike" until more appropriate approaches are allowed to develop.

REFERENCES

1. Ambulatory health care in the city of Boston: needs, resources, and priorities, prepared for the Office of Region I, Department of Health, Education, and Welfare, Cambridge, Mass., 1974, Abt Associates.
2. Branch, L. G.: Understanding the health and social service needs of people over age 65, report submitted in partial fulfillment of grants 90-A-641/01 and 90-A-641/02, Washington, D.C., 1977, Administration on Aging, Department of Health, Education, and Welfare.
3. Brody, E.: Long-term care for the elderly: optimums, options, and opportunities, J. Am. Geriatr. Soc. **19**:432, 1971.
4. Department of Health, Education, and Welfare: Vital and health statistics estimates from National Health Interview Survey, United States, 1972, series 10, no. 85, Washington, D.C., 1973, the Department.
5. Dorsey, J.: Physician distribution in Boston and Brookline, 1940-1969, Med. Care **7**:429-439, 1969.
6. Feltin, M.: Community-based home care, paper presented before the American Public Health Association, Washington, D.C., Nov., 1977.
7. Frank, K.: Government support of nursing home care, N. Engl. J. Med. **287**:538, 1972.
8. Kirk, E.: Personal communication regarding the three-year experience of the Uphams Corner Health Center, community-based home care program emplying homemaker/home health aides.
9. McLaughlin, L.: House calls in the inner city, Boston Globe, April 27, 1978, p. 3.
10. Mark, R. L., Willemain, T. R., and Master, R. J.: Nursing home telemedicine project final report, NSF/RA 76-0282, Division of Advanced Productivity Research and Technology, Boston, July, 1976, National Science Foundation.

11. Master, R.: Coping with regulations in long-term care, Symposium on Long-Term Care, Oct., 1978, University of Massachusetts, In press.
12. National Center for Health Statistics: Characteristics of residents in institutions for the aged and chronically ill in the United States, April-June, 1963, series 12, no. 2, Washington, D.C., 1965, Department of Health, Education, and Welfare.
13. National Center for Health Statistics: Current estimates from health interview survey in the United States, 1970, series 10, no. 72, Washington, D.C., Department of Health, Education, and Welfare.
14. Rosenberg, C. E.: The hospital in America: a century's perspective, Philadelphia, 1971, American Philosophical Library, pp. 181-196.
15. Solon, J. A.: Medical care: its social and organizational aspects. Nursing homes and medical care, N. Engl. J. Med. **268**:1067, 1963.
16. Tomich, J. H.: The expanded role of the nurse: current status and future prospects in the nursing profession: view through the mist, New York, 1978, McGraw-Hill Book Co., pp.299-307.
17. Trager, B.: Home health services in the United States, Washington, D.C., 1972, Department of Health, Education, and Welfare.

CHAPTER 11

Discharge planning: a clinical dietitian's perspective

PATRICIA M. KEARNEY
PATRICIA GLEASON-CLAYDON

Food and nutrition are integral parts of our life cycle. A physiologic necessity, food is the essence of life. It may also be symbolic of status, wealth, virility, love, affection, masculinity, femininity, security, religiousness, reward, or enjoyment. We use food for communication or as a means for control through acceptance or rejection. The rebellious rehabilitation patient, the anorexic patient, the pregnant teenager dismaybed by her body image, and the depressed elderly patient who has undergone enviromental changes may express their fears, frustrations, and anger by refusing nourishment. The cachectic cancer patient, a helpless victim of disease, may grasp at the opportunity to try supplemental feedings to aid in self-treatment. Ingestion of food may be the one constant factor that a patient can hold onto during a time of tumult and uncertainty. The patient may then shift from passively receiving care to actively participating in the treatment, thus achieving some level of self-sufficiency and autonomy.

This transition is a complex process. All biomedical, physical, social, and personal factors that characterize each individual's living environment must be identified when the discharge planning process is initiated after admission to a health care facility. It is the dietitian's responsibility to utilize the information obtained from an analysis of these environmental factors and to develop a comprehensive care plan that can be followed by the patient and the other multidisciplinary team members.

The professional role of the dietitian is an active one in terms of interaction with both the patient and other multidisciplinary team members. All remain accountable to the patient for delivering optimum health care. In an organized discharge planning process, the curative and educational components of care should start immediately. The five basic steps, assessment, diagnosis, prescription, implementation, and evaluation, are common to all the disciplines and provide a methodical and dynamic means for the delivery of health care.

ROLE OF THE CLINICAL DIETITIAN IN DISCHARGE PLANNING

The delivery of quality nutritional care has necessitated the expansion of the clinical dietitian's role. Early dietitians were generalists primarily concerned with diet management and the art of feeding people. This role was expanded as the science of human nutrition demanded that a dietitian assess nutritional status, identify problems, and plan and administer nutritional care to patients in various life situations.[1]

The clinical dietitian, as the person accountable for the nutritional health of the patient, must assume the responsibility of becoming an independent decision maker and an agent for behavioral change. No longer is it possible for the dietitian to remain in a physician-oriented role, performing technical skills as prescribed by the physician's order book. Clinical dietitians should actively determine their role in the health care setting rather than passively reacting to the dictates of other health professionals. Foster[2] describes the type A dietitian as one who is responsible and accountable for patient care and takes initiative when dealing with professional peers. The type B dietitian responds adequately when called upon to adapt diet orders to patients' needs but basically remains passive in a professional role. These categories can be applied to all professionals. The goal of discharge planning and the health care team is to provide optimum patient care, and it can be accomplished by type A professionals composing a type A team. It is the clinical dietitian's professional responsibility and obligation to both the patient and the team not only to respond when called upon but to seek out pertinent information and inform the team of its importance. In a type A team the interations depend greatly on mutual support and referral. Each member must be aware of what the others' roles entail. A lack of up-to-date knowledge may lead to inappropriate referrals or patient care planning. Each discipline is responsible for making a unique and specialized contribution to the patient care plan. This capability renders each team member indispensable.

CLINICAL DIETITIAN'S ACCOUNTABILITY TO THE PATIENT

The clinical dietitian is accountable to the patient for delivering optimum nutritional care. Short-term restorative care and long-term continuous care are two prime concerns.

Mechanisms for implementing a comprehensive plan including discharge planning should be initiated during the patient's admission to the hospital and should be continued after discharge. There are four fundamental environments to consider in a comprehensive study of a patient's life situation. These environmental factors are important in determining various components of a patient care plan.

1. *Biomedical environment:* past medical and nutritional history, present med-

ical and nutritional status, anthropometric measurements, laboratory data, test results, treatment procedures, medications

2. *Physical environment:* living situation, available material resources (financial, transportation, food), available supportive services
3. *Social environment:* cultural habits, ethnic background, peers, family, occupation, religion, recreation
4. *Personal environment:* level of education, learning ability, learning preferences, self-perception, motivation, goals, self-evaluation patterns, childhood experiences, psychological makeup

The nutritional care plan leading to discharge should consider the above factors and isolate those that are most significant. Logical, methodical steps should then be carefully planned. The patient education process and the establishment of ongoing support structures should be initiated at the time of the patient's admission. The health care facility is a learning center, and the patient participates in a "live-in" course. The community and nutritional follow-up provided for in the discharge plan serve as the "refresher" courses. The discharge plan is the course outline and should ensure a comprehensive learning experience. An integrated plan will reinforce the patient's education in as many ways as possible. The dietitian must be responsible for keeping the discharge planning team informed of the nutritional considerations concerning the patient and for educating both the patient and significant other persons involved in supporting the patient on a long-term basis. All care participants should be informed about the rationale underlying therapy, treatment, instructional tools, and resources available for delivering quality nutritional care.

DISCHARGE PLANNING PROCESS

The overall goal of discharge planning is to bring the patient to the optimum level of health and help the patient maintain that status. Restorative care and the development of support structures for health maintenance can be facilitated through an organized discharge planning process. The assessment, diagnosis, prescription, implementation, and evaluation procedures offer an organized means for providing care. These five steps of the discharge planning process provide a systematic method that offers a common approach for all disciplines. Individually, each step has a specific and functional purpose; together the steps provide for a continuous flow of care and enhance the ongoing process, as the chart on p. 133 shows.

Assessment

A thorough assessment of the patient's nutritional status provides a basis for appropriate counseling and optimum nutritional care. Factual data concerning the patient's status may be obtained by taking a comprehensive view of the patient's four fundamental environments, as previously discussed. The exploration of these environments may be accomplished by using the following accessible methods of data collection.

FLOW OF DISCHARGE PLANNING

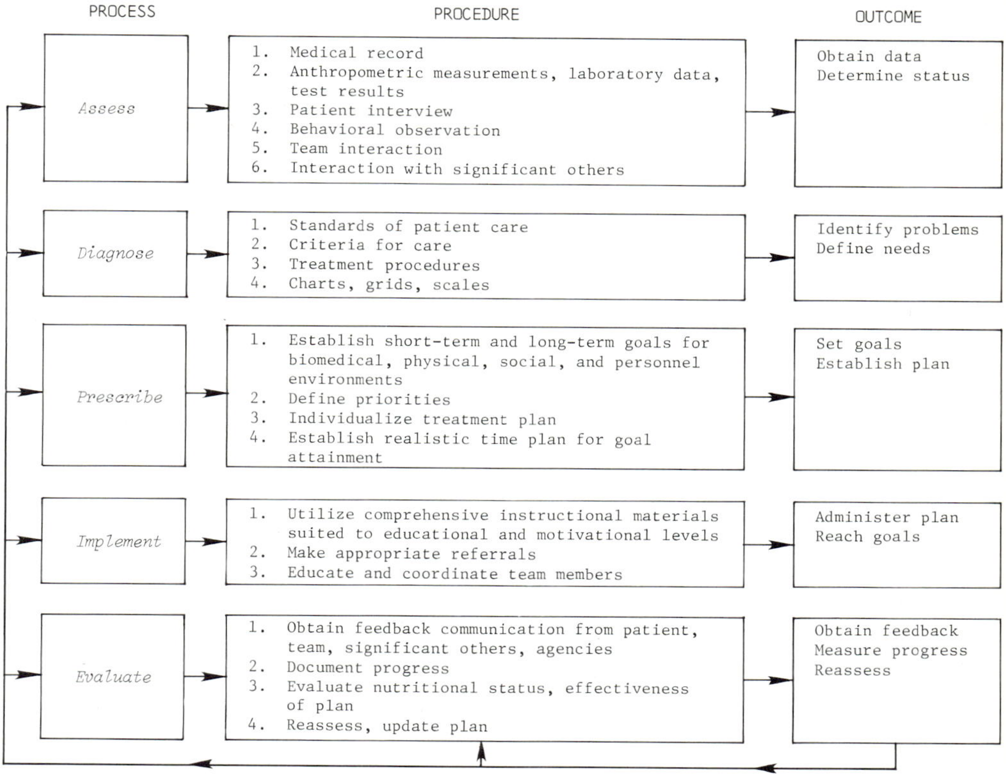

Medical record. The medical record provides documented data and pertinent information concerning the patient's present and past medical history, laboratory work, anthropometric measurements, tests and procedures, medications, and emotional and social status.

Patient interview. The patient interview provides additional subjective data concerning the patient's life-style, living situation, cultural and recreational habits, eating habits, food tolerances, estimated caloric intake (dietary history), and self-perception and motivation in relation to present health status.

Discussing food and eating patterns is often a nonthreatening way for the patient to disclose pertinent information about his life-style in terms of the social, physical, and personal environments.

Daily observations. Daily observations provide an opportunity for an ongoing assessment process by which to evaluate compliance while the patient is in the hospital. In addition, a continuous reassessment of the treatment plan can be made.

Team interaction. A continuous flow of knowledge and support is made possible through team interaction.

Data collection. Another viable means of communication is the use of a single data collection form. Assessment data as well as information pertaining to the patient's diagnosis, care plan prescription, implementation format, and continued evaluation are recorded in a concise manner. The form serves as a useful tool in the continuous assessment process. It is useful for keeping accurate, well-outlined records of the patient's treatments, medications, medical and nutritional status, and progress, as well as serving as a quick reference for correlating and using the data. Placed in a notebook or on a clipboard, the form is easily accessible at rounds or while visiting the patients. It can also be used as a reference for other members of the health care team if it is left in an accessible location such as the nursing station.

The use of this type of form does not eliminate the necessity of recording pertinent information in the medical record. It merely provides the dietitian with an information-gathering device that may be shared with others when appropriate.

The analysis of the data that have been collected during the assessment process is a crucial element in the overall outcome of the care that is to be provided. In the absence of pertinent information the dietitian should initiate the appropriate tests, laboratory or anthropometric orders or both, and procedures that are needed to make the assessment complete.

Diagnosis

The diagnosis identifies the problems and defines specific patient needs. During this process a diagnostic statement can be made in which the patient's overall health and nutritional status is delineated. Problem identification and definition of the patient's needs should be explicit and provide a sound basis for the diagnosis. Before any diagnosis can be established, the problems identified within the patient's biomedical, physical, social, and personal environments must be considered and their impact on the patient's nutritional status determined.

To make appropriate diagnostic decisions and requests, the dietitian needs to have knowledge of the patient's disease pathology, laboratory work, medications, pyschosocial history, and other multidisciplinary involvement. The relationship of drugs to diet is one area where a diagnostic problem may be identified. The interactions between certain drugs and foods may affect the nutritional status of the patient. For example, certain medications taken in combination with food substances may act as appetite depressants, irritate the gastric mucosa, influence the bacterial flora in the intestines, or directly affect absorption.[3] Laboratory data and the various test and treatment procedures that the patient undergoes while in the hospital are crucial tools in diagnosing nutritional status as well as in providing care.

The patient who goes for a test each morning before breakfast and who routinely returns late presents the team with a problem. Often only a small snack is given when a patient returns just before lunch. In this case the patient has missed a vital part of treatment-nourishment. Communicating this type of data will enable the dietitian to correlate intake with weight changes and consequently influence the scheduling of the patient's test or treatment plan.

Various tools may be developed to aid the dietitian in making a nutritional

EATING SCORE GRID

Eating scores

1--Density fluids
2--Density fluids
3--Picking
4--Starches/desserts
5--Entree only
6--1/2 or more of each item
7--All*

DATE	EATING SCORE	CARE LEVEL	DIS-ORIENTED	POSI-TIVE	ANXIOUS, ANGRY	FATIGUED, DEPRESSED	N/V	N/A	COMMENTS

*Prepared by the Clinical Staff, Department of Dietetics and Nutrition, The Brigham and Women's Hospital, Boston.

diagnosis. One such tool is the eating score grid shown above. By using this type of recording mechanism, the dietitian can observe the patient's eating schedule and mood changes and make a correlation when necessary. This information provides the dietitian with additional data for diagnosis and is a useful tool that can be shared with the other team members to provide a focal point for care (e.g., an obese individual may eat when depressed or the cancer patient may not eat at all after radiation treatment). Both the dietitian and the members of other disciplines will be able to use such information to provide better care. The eating score grid is especially useful to the dietitian who is helping to determine the level of nutritional care needed. It can be helpful in identifying those patients who presumably do not appear at nutritional risk and is also useful in categorizing patients according to certain levels. The levels that are established will dictate frequency of intervention by the dietitian. For example, a level 1 patient is someone who enters the hospital without any apparent nutritional deficiencies and maintains an eating score of seven when evaluated on a regular basis. This person may be seen by a nutrition support person (e.g., a diet technician or aide), with occasional intervention by the dietitian. Levels 2 and 3 are those patients needing moderate intervention, and Levels 4 and 5 are those needing intense intervention on a regular basis.

Correlating those factors presented in the physical, social, and personal environments is a vital element of the diagnostic procedure. The living situation to which a person will be returning, ethnic and religious implications, learning capabilities of the patient or significant others, and a patient's motivational level are all influential in the diagnostic procedure.

Prescription

The nutrition prescription and care plan set goals and establish organized means with which to reach those goals. Both short- and long-term goals must promote the patient's assumption of maximum responsibility for his own health. The prescription should address the biomedical, physical, social, and personal environments of the patient. Using this information, the dietitian can formulate a specific nutitional prescription, including a diet prescription. Sequential steps for goal attainment may be established. It is emphasized that a nutrition prescription is an important component of the patient care plan, even when a modified diet order is not indicated.

An effective nutritional prescription depends on the plan's appropriateness in addressing the motivational level and needs of the patient as well as on the capabilities of the team to support the plan. The overall goal is to establish a workable plan for, and most importantly *with*, the patient. This plan should take the patient through hospitalization, on to an extended care facility if necessary, and subsequently to discharge home. In establishing the nutritional care plan, the dietitian must often solicit the help of the patient's family and friends as well as that of the other team members, especially if a special bonding has already been established.

When a nutritional prescription or plan is formulated, short- and long-term goals are set with the patient or significant others or both. These goals should be individualized so that they can become useful tools in the education process. For the plan to be effective, the patient should be informed of the expected outcome and should be aware of the stages of progression as they are reached. It is essential for good nutitional care and discharge planning that patients take an active part in their therapy at the first sign that they are progressing out of the critical stage of their condition. However, in most instances the dietitian should not wait for patients to verbalize their desires or interests. The assessment and diagnostic steps should provide sufficient information to establish the basis for a care plan. It is the dietitian's and the other team members' responsibility to try to motivate the patient to move from a passive state to active participation in the care plan. The patient then becomes personally accountable.

To be effective, a nutrition care plan must be developed according to the situational as well as the factual data. Where the patient is coming from should always be kept in mind. The cachectic cancer patient who in instructed to increase daily protein and caloric intake to remain well nourished and in a state of positive nitrogen balance may very often be met with problems associated with the cancer and treatment regimen. In addition to the side effects (nausea, anorexia, vomiting, and diarrhea) that so often accompany cancer therapy, there may be financial limitations that lend themselves to increased anxiety. In such situations it may be necessary to place the patient on a supplemental feeding regimen until there is improvement in nutritional status. Simultaneously the dietitian and the social worker can be working out a program for situational and financial assistance.

The inadequate availability of personnel in most health care facilities often makes it necessary for the dietitian to make an objective decision based on which of the patients receiving care need intense intervention and which ones can be handled by nutrition support personnel. Standards that define the quality of care to be given to patients may serve as a basis for the nutritional prescription.

Specific criteria for reaching these standards must be established and not left merely to the discretion of the individual health professional. The criteria should be founded on professional expertise and professional literature[4] and should be relevant, understandable, measurable, behavioral, and achievable. Process criteria measure the appropriateness of treatment and the procedures used to reach a certain goal with a patient. Outcome criteria measure the quality of short or long-term results. Thus the patient has the right to quality care based on optimum standards focused on individual needs.

When the dietitian develops a discharge care plan, it is necessary to keep in mind the type of extended or ambulatory care that the patient will be receiving. Test and treatment procedures that are undergone on an ambulatory basis also present a nutritional problem for certain patients (e.g., the cancer patient receiving radiation thereapy, the renal patient on dialysis, or the arthritic patient coming in for physical thereapy). Specific plans should be developed to assist the patient when therapy interferes with normal daily routines and dietary patterns.

Implementation

The implementation phase of discharge planning involves administering the prescription to reach the stated goals. Whereas the prescription establishes the "what" of therapy, the implementation must define the "how." Specific workable recommendations and assignments must be given. Mechanisms for the continuance of care should be initiated by developing support structures in the patient's immediate environment as well as in the future environment.

Implementation of the prescription involves administering patient care services, collecting data, participating in team interaction, and educating the patient. Included in patient care services is the delivery of palatable and appropriate meals and nourishment. Current data that document a patient's status within the four fundamental environments (previously discussed) must be collected and compiled. Pertinent information should be accessible to all care providers.

Implementation of a discharge plan for each patient involves combining the efforts of the patient, the patient's family, and all members of the team. Team interaction and communication are vital to the implementation process. Each member of the team either proceeds in the role of facilitator or remains in the background as an adviser or consultant. It is important to remember that all interactions with the patient should yield support for the ongoing plan of care. All disciplines should work together to keep each member of the team informed as to the patient's progress, areas of concern, and need for additional assistance. The communication between team members might be as basic as the nurse's informing the dietary

PATIENT EDUCATION DOCUMENTATION

DATE	Subject	PROVIDER	*PT education evaluation*
	Confirmation of diet		
	Initial nutritional assessment		
	Change of diet recommendation		
	Status report (every 7 days minimum)		
	Transfer summary/ discharge report		

Instruction material used: Booklet_____ Sheet_____ Other_____

Title of instructional materials:_____

Instruction given: Patient _____ Spouse _____ Significant other _____

Diet:_____

Seven steps of education

DATE	Subject	PROVIDER	*D/C planning*
	Rationale in relation to disease		DCS_____ CC_____ VNA_____
	Develop meal plan with patient or family		Other _____
	Give instruction material		
	Discuss evaluation of selective menu choices		
	Discuss dining out		
	Discuss marketing food options		
	Discuss food labeling		

*Prepared by the Clinical Staff, Department of Dietetics and Nutrition, The Brigham and Women's Hospital, Boston.

department when inappropriate food items have appeared on a patient's tray. It could also be as detailed as when a nursing home is visited by a dietitian and is found to be incapable of providing the patient with the necessary nutritional support. Each discipline should be aware of the Department of Dietetics and Nutrition's Standards of Patient Care, as well as the criteria that have been developed to guide nutrition staff members as they provide optimum nutritional care in the process of treating patients and planning for an appropriate discharge site. Progress notes, daily floor rounds, and one-to-one consultation are effective means of daily communication, and participation in the multidisciplinary audit facilitates effective group input and evaluation of care.

The dietitian's role as an educator is important to the successful implementation of nutritional care. The dietitian who once was the didactic instructor relating the technicalities of giving a specified diet must now become an agent for behavioral change. The patient must be taught the what, how, and why of therapy and must then be motivated to follow the plan through hospitalization to placement in extended care facility or a return home. At some point during the implementation phase, patients must realize their role and responsibility for their own health care. Patient involvement is a key factor in successful patient education. The more functions that patients will perform—keeping records of daily intake, selecting a menu from the hospital menu or making appropriate choices from a restaurant menu while keeping within the diet prescription—the greater the patient's participation and involvement. This approach reinforces and enhances knowledge and hopefully increases a patient's willingness to comply. It also enables the dietitian to evaluate when some of the learning tasks must be retraced and thus relearned. Educational materials should be geared toward the patient's educational and motivational capacities. Appropriate learning materials can be adapted to meet a patient's level of sophistication. There is no age barrier when it comes to instructional tools, and the use of nutrition-related games, coloring books, or quizzes is often more effective than a detailed diet sheet in persuading the disenchanted patient to become involved. These tools may also prove to be useful for other disciplines (e.g., occupational therapy, social service, or nursing).

Working with other disciplines to develop multipurpose educational materials is also useful. The pharmacist and dietitian together can produce appropriate pamphlets to inform patients about their medications and the effects that certain foods may have on either drug or nutrient utilization. The social worker and the dietitian may collaborate to foster patient participation in educational support programs offered by the community after discharge.

Patient education must be initiated during hospitalization. An organized approach to patient education and care documentation is important (p. 138).

Evaluation

The evaluation process must provide a mechanism for measuring progress, reassessing the patient's needs, and updating the prescription and its implementation. The process should involve continuous detailed documentation that can be utilized for feedback communication and in patient care audits. The patient should be directly involved with his own evaluation and reevaluation. Both oral and written methods of evaluation may be used. When this process is consciously started in the hospital, it is more probable that the patient's self-diagnostic and evaluative skills will be utilized after discharge.

Feedback from family members, referral agencies, or extended care facilities is important. A patient who has been placed on a restrictive diet or one who has undergone a procedure that has altered his capacity to handle food should not be discharged from the hospital without some type of accessible support structure. Referring the patient to a neighborhood health center or outpatient clinic to see a nutritionist, or making a referral to a community agency (e.g., a visiting nurse association or an extension service of the Department of Agriculture) when assistance can be given, will ensure continuous care. Feedback from these agencies is a useful evaluation tool. Some agencies have their own forms that ask for a copy of the discharge diet and a description of the care the patient has received. However, not all service-based agencies that provide more practical assistance (food preparation, shopping, and budgetary tips) rather than medical assistance have a standard referral form or method of providing feedback. The development of a formal referral form would assist an extended care agency as well as the referring institution. It would provide the agency with some general information about the patient's care and give the referring institution a means of obtaining an updated report on the patient's progress and an evaluation of the patient's response to the service. This information should be filed in the patient's record so that it remains accessible.

CLINICAL DIETITIAN AS A MEMBER OF A MULTIDISCIPLINARY TEAM

An efficiently operating health care team must always have a coordinator to compile, sort, and appropriately redistribute information for discharge. The coordinator of this comprehensive data base may be a regularly designated health team member (e.g., the primary care nurse, who has 24-hour patient care accountability) or another health team member whose expertise predominates in the care of a particular patient. The patient may also designate a leader by establishing close rapport and a sense of trust with one particular team member.

When each team member's role is determined in response to the needs of the patient and the needs of the other disciplines, the services provided are of greater value to all. Team dynamics have three commonalities: people, interation, and change. The team comprises the patient as well as all involved health professionals. When the team members' roles are mutually accommodating rather than isolated, the interations fulfill needs, influence one another's care, and increase the efficacy of therapy through reinforcement. A dynamic group is active and changing. The goal of a discharge planning team is to initiate and maintain dynamic interaction among disciplines to facilitate the most effective and efficient strategy for bringing a patient to the highest health potential.

Team dynamics, filtered through the coordinator, should dictate whether the dietitian will (1) act as the primary care provider, (2) provide consultation, or (3) receive consultation from another provider. Nutritional intervention may be the cornerstone of therapy for diet-controlled diabetic patients, anorectic patients, geriatric patients with poor dentition, and patients having such problems as food intolerances or allergies, malabsorption syndrome, or gastrointestinal distress. The dietitian may consult with the occupational therapist who is working with a patient

EXCHANGE OF NUTRITIONAL SERVICES

Clinical dietitian	Physician	Patient
Relate specifics of:	*Relate specifics of:*	*Benefits from:*
Diet therapy	Disease pathology	Appropriate diet
Recommended diet modification	Progress/update	Updated diet therapy
Patient's compliance	Effectiveness of therapy	Individualized nutrition care plan
Food-drug interactions	Medications	Effective medication
Rationale for nutritionally indicated laboratory tests	Rationale, results for laboratory tests	Comprehensive assessment
Implications of tests/treatment on dietary intake	Rationale, implications of treatment	Appropriate scheduling (frequency, timing)

Clinical dietitian	Nurse	Patient
Relate specifics of:	*Relate specifics of:*	*Benefits from:*
Therapeutic diet	Appropriateness of diet	Appropriate care
Patient's preferences	Patient's preferences	Acknowledgment of patient's input
Patient's tolerance	Patient's tolerance	Relief
Therapy for complications with nutritional implications	Existing complications (e.g., nausea, constipation)	Updated care
Laboratory data	Laboratory results	Efficiency, effectiveness
Test/treatment procedures	Test/treatment scheduling	Individualized care
Allergies	Allergies	Effective medication
Food-drug interactions	Medications	Effectiveness, efficiency
Food delivery procedures	Accuracy of food services	Accurate and appropriate foods

Clinical dietitian	Social worker	Patient
Relate specifics of:	*Relate specifics of:*	*Benefits from:*
Therapeutic diet	Patient's perception of diet therapy	Reinforcement; needs are better understood
Implications of physical environment: information on available resources (food, nutrition education, community services, support groups)	Need for referral, coordinated services	
Implications of social environment: peer pressure/support, family pressure/support, life-style change	Social situation	Appropriate care plan
Implications of personal environment: body image, mood swings, attitude, prior experiences	Patient's perception of self, living situation	Appropriate care plan
Nutritional intervention	Need for crisis intervention	Immediate needs addressed
Nutritional expertise in group setting	Dynamics of group therapy	Group reinforcement, support

Clinical dietitian	Physical therapist	Patient
Relate specifics of:	*Relate specifics of:*	*Benefits from:*
Therapeutic diet: diabetic controls, meal pattern	Exercise schedule: energy needs, need for supplementation	Synchronized plan (appropriate meal/snack pattern)
Treatment for weight control	Design for appropriate activity schedule	Reinforced treatment
Nutritional therapy for behavior modification	Exercise plan for behavior modification	Comprehensive care
Appropriate laboratory data (e.g., serum levels)	Energy requirements for exercise routine	Appropriate care

Continued.

EXCHANGE OF NUTRITIONAL SERVICES—CONT'D

Clinical dietitian	Occupational therapist	Patient
Relate specifics of:	*Relate specifics of:*	*Benefits from:*
Therapeutic diet	Patient's physical limitations, tolerances	Personalized care
Possible foods to accommodate nutritional, mechanical needs	Ability to use utensils	Personalized care
Appropriate foods	Ability to swallow, ingest food	Personalized care

Clinical dietitian	Extended care provider	Patient
Relate specifics of:	*Relate specifics of:*	*Benefits from:*
Requirements for continued implementation of care plan	Feasibility of continuing care plan (e.g., TPN, special food preparation)	Appropriate referral
Therapeutic diet	Feedback on patient's compliance, tolerance, progress	Continuance of care
Nutrition care plan modification	Indications for modifications in nutrition care plan	Updated therapy

Clinical dietitian	Hospital administrator	Patient
Relate specifics of:	*Relate specifics of:*	*Benefits from:*
Statistical data: type and amount of services, cost effectiveness, personnel needed to provide quality patient care	Availability of adequate resources: space, support third-party reimbursement, budget	Increased availability of quality services
Professional participation in decision-making process	Obtaining positions on decision-making boards and medical review committees	Representation of nutritional needs

with dysphagia. Consultation may be sought from the physician when additional knowledge concerning the pathophysiology of a disease state is needed. The mutual support that team members offer one another results in higher-quality care for the patient, as indicated by the chart on exchange of nutritional services (pp. 141-142).

Since limitations of a process are often sorted out only after the process has begun, there is a need for effective feedback mechanisms. Throughout the assessment, diagnostic, prescriptive, implementation, and evaluation processes, it is important that each member of the team report to the dietitian pertinent subjective and objective data concerning the patient's nutritional prescription, care plan, and overall compliance. Careful documentation provides not only an effective means of interdisciplinary communication but an ongoing record of the patient care services provided. Interdisciplinary communication is a vital factor in effective team interaction. Sound lines of communication improve

- Knowledge about the patient
- Efficacy of services
- Planning and coordination
- Cohesiveness of the team
- Competence of health professionals

The expanded pool of knowledge about the patient better enables the team to formulate a personal discharge plan. The efficacy of services may be greatly improved through cooperation. Acquiring a weight measurement on a regular basis may pose problems for the dietitian who cannot move a disabled patient; however, the physical therapist could walk or wheel a patient to the scale during an exercise session and thus perform a twofold service. Changes in a patient's weight will then become more meaningful to the physical therapist when they are discussed at rounds. Such coordination of effort helps the team to become a more cohesive group in which individual goals are integrated into the team's goals and a unified purpose is promoted.

Communication strategies provide the means for the reciprocal exchange of ideas and services. Formalized meetings and rounds allow team members to update, reevaluate, and test progressive ideas for the patient care plan. Informal oral communication is vital to the more immediate processing of care. The following case study will demonstrate how the clinical dietitian assesses the patient's biomedical, physical, social, and personal environments. It will also illustrate the interactions of the team in providing a comprehensive discharge plan.

CASE STUDY

M. J. is a 66-year-old woman who was in a state of impending hepatic coma at the time of her admission.

Biomedical environment

M. J. has no significant past medical history, with the exception of a hysterectomy 17 years prior to admission. The patient was transferred from a community hospital and presented with a diagnosis of (1) Laennec's cirrhosis, (2) edema, (3) aortic stenosis, (4) hyperaldosteronism, and (5) severe hypokalemia. Her symptoms included jaundice, ascites, fever, diarrhea, hypertension, abdominal distension and pain, fatigue, anorexia, anemia, splenomegaly, gastrointestinal bleeding, and liver flap.

The patient had no known nutritional deficiencies prior to this illness. She had supplemented her diet with multivitamins for several years. Up until one year ago the patient's weight (80 kg, 175 lb) was 35% above her ideal weight for her height (167 cm, 5 ft 6 in.) and stature. Over the previous nine months the patient had experienced a weight loss of 13.5 kg (30 lb), with an additional 6.75 kg (15 lb) weight loss secondary to anorexia, nausea, and vomiting during the previous six weeks.

The initial laboratory values showed the following:

T. bilirubin, 8.2%
Albumin, 1.9
Prothrombin time, 38%
Glucose, 131 mg/dl
Serum alkaline phosphatase, 180 mU/dl
SGOT, 100 mU/dl
LDH, 260
BUN, 72
BP, 160/90

Test results presented further implications. X-ray films showed the presence of esophageal varices, and hepatic scanning indicated the presence of splenomegaly. There were ECG changes that showed S-T segment changes in all leads with unifocal premature ventricular contractions (PVCs). Folate, potassium chloride, aluminum hydroxide gel (Amphojel), multivitamins, Kaopectate, and thiamine were administered.

Physical environment

M. J. has lived alone in a small, single-family dwelling in a rural area since the death of her husband 9 months ago. Although she is a Medicaid recipient, she does not use any other form of social or community support. She is able to maintain a moderate standard of living on her husband's pension.

Social environment

Subsequent to her husband's death, M. J. became progressively lonelier. She lessened her church and social activities and began drinking alone to excess. Her only ongoing relationship was with her one married daughter, who lived 50 miles away. Prior to her seclusion, she and her husband had enjoyed dining out and playing cards with friends.

Personal environment

M. J. is a high school graduate without further formal education, with the exception of one course in needlework several years ago. The patient was reported to have been known as a heavy drinker during her youth, although during her married life she was classified as a social drinker.

Discussion

Biomedically, the patient appeared to be in acute distress. Conditions presenting in her physical, social, and personal environments appeared to be causative factors in the etiology of her present situation. Living alone, in self-imposed exclusion from social outlets, appeared to promote M. J.'s sense of loneliness and depression. The result was an excessive consumption of alcohol along with a declining nutritional state.

A primary diagnosis of impending hepatic coma, multiple medical and nutritional complications, and a poor psychosocial situation indicated that intensive intervention by all team members was needed. A comprehensive care plan was developed by the team to help M. J. make the transition from apathy to active and interested participation in her own health care. The admitting physician initiated the appropriate medical intervention. Due to the severity of the hepatic condition and other medical complications, the prescribed diet focused on a low-protein, low-sodium, soft diet with a daily fluid restriction. These diet restrictions were gradually eased as the patient's biomedical condition improved. As improvement progressed, the patient's physical, social, and personal environments could be addressed more fully.

The patient, patient's daughter, dietitian, and social worker were able to work out plans for a viable living situation. She would live temporarily with her daughter until arrangements could be made for her to move into a senior citizens' residential complex. This site would provide her with a means for socialization through various functions and the elderly lunch program (Title VII). Arrangements were made for her to be visited initially by a visiting nurse. Due to her present nutritional status and her expressed interest in weight maintenance, follow-up visits to the outpatient nutritionist were also scheduled. Working with the dietitian, the physical therapist was able to support M. J.'s weight maintenance program by developing an appropriate exercise regimen.

The occupational therapist worked with the patient to renew her interest in her crewel work and other outside activities.

During hospitalization, difficulties with the patient's noncompliance in taking several medications were reported by the primary nurse. It was decided that a single prenatal multivitamin that included folic acid would be sufficient.

Prior to her discharge the team reviewed M. J.'s case. In view of the new support structures established in her living situation, it was felt that alcohol ingestion would not be a continued problem; however, intervention with the social worker was planned.

M. J. was discharged from the hospital four weeks after admission with defined goals and objectives and a concrete plan with which to attain these goals.

SUMMARY

It is essential for good patient care and a complete discharge care plan that all members of the multidisciplinary team interact with each other. The clinical dietitian is responsible for the nutritional health of the patient and acts as a resource person for the other disciplines as well.

The flow of the discharge care plan as it relates to the four fundamental environmental factors takes the patient from the first day of institutionalization through the course of care and back into the community.

REFERENCES

1. Forcier, J. D., Kight, M. A., and Sheehan, E. T.: Point of view: acculturation in clinical dietetics, J. Am. Diet. Assoc. **70**:181, 1977.
2. Foster, J. T.: A hospital administrator's view of the shared responsibility, J. Am. Diet. Assoc. **67**:539, 1975.
3. Hospital pharmacy "white sheet," Columbus, Ohio, 1970, Philips Roxane Laboratories.
4. Walters, F. M., and Crumley, S. J., editors: Patient care audit: a quality assurance procedure manual for dietitians, Chicago, 1978, American Dietetic Association.

ADDITIONAL READINGS

American Dietetic Association: The dietitian in primary health care, J. Am. Diet. Assoc. **70**:157, 1977.

Baumgarten, S., and Collins, M. E.: The dietitian in continuing care, J. Am. Diet. Assoc. **67**:576, 1975.

Mahoney, M. J., and Cagginla, A. W.: Applying behavioral methods to nutrition counseling, J. Am. Diet. Assoc. **72**:372, 1978.

Mason, M., Wenberb, B., and Welsch, P. K.: The dynamics of clinical dietetics, New York, 1977, John Wiley & Sons.

Thiele, M. C., and Hankin, J. H.: Training nutritionists for comprehensive health delivery system, J. Am. Diet. Assoc. **70**:189, 1977.

Wade, J. E.: Role of a clinical dietitian specialist on a nutrition support service, J. Am. Diet. Assoc. **70**:185, 1977.

Weed, J. E., and Mallenson, A.: Establishing guidelines for peer review of the clinical dietitian, J. Am. Diet. Assoc. **70**:157, 1977.

Zifferblatt, S. M., and Wilbur, C. S.: Dietary counseling: some realistic expections and guidelines, J. Am. Diet. Assoc. **72**:372, 1978.

CHAPTER 12

Discharge planning: a physical therapist's perspective

JEAN OULUND PETEET

The physical therapist provides services in a multiplicity of settings: private practice, home health agencies, acute care and chronic care facilities, rehabilitation hospitals, nursing homes, outpatient facilities, and school systems. The therapist plans and administers treatment programs for patients of all ages to restore function, relieve pain, and prevent disability after disease, injury, or loss of body parts. The physical therapist's role in discharge planning is not the same in all settings. In the acute setting the therapist provides or supervises direct care but also frequently serves as a consultant when it becomes necessary to recommend long-term physical therapy. In the rehabilitation hospital the therapist is intensively involved in direct care *and* in planning for complex discharge needs. In the outpatient setting the therapist usually provides direct care. However, the setting may be somewhat isolated, requiring extra effort to coordinate treatment. In all settings it is imperative that the physical therapist become part of multidisciplinary team. The team may consist of only the therapist and physician or may involve numerous other health professionals. This chapter will discuss the therapist's role in discharge planning. General guidelines and principles will be provided, and specific suggestions for implementing the process of discharge from the acute hospital, rehabilitation facility, nursing home, or outpatient setting will be discussed. The chapter will conclude with a discussion of the therapist's role in evaluating the discharge process.

GENERAL PRINCIPLES OF DISCHARGE PLANNING

Quality discharge planning should begin at the time of admission. There are five general characteristics needed by the physical therapist for participation in discharge planning:

1. Commitment to, and ability to plan for, patient and family involvement

2. Ability to provide clear and objective chart documentation, including short and long-term goals from admission to discharge
3. Understanding of regulatory requirements as they relate to reimbursement for patient services
4. Knowledge of the availability of community services and general insurance coverage (e.g., for patient equipment)
5. Clear understanding of the roles of licensed physical therapists, physical therapist assistants, aides, and other health team members, to facilitate appropriate delegation of responsibility

Regulatory requirements for physical therapy involvement in discharge planning are presently written in general terms. The standards of practice developed by the American Physical Therapy Association are similarly general, but they are helpful in giving therapists a framework for involvement in discharge planning. The therapist is expected to use professional judgment in "planning the patient's program, implementing and supervising that program, evaluating and changing that program, maintaining adequate records of the case, and filing appropriate progress reports with the attending physician." Furthermore, "it is the responsibility of the physical therapist to inform the referring practitioner when, in his judgment, the patient cannot benefit from treatment."[1] Undoubtedly, guidelines will become more specific as regulatory agencies continue to seek means of cost control. Physical therapists should welcome and search for opportunities to develop and maintain guidelines for discharge planning that can ensure both cost control and quality care.

Teamwork is essential in discharge planning in all settings but is often difficult to achieve. Frustrations usually center around staff-to-staff conflicts, rather than patient-to-staff conflicts. One frequently hears such remarks as, "I just can't get nursing to follow through with sliding board transfers with the patient so that the patient can go home wheelchair independent," or "Why can't the physician understand that we have no more to offer this patient?" No simple or quick formulas exist to resolve these conflicts. A willingness to share concerns with other team members and, if appropriate, to acknowledge reponsibility for helping to create conflicts is needed. Once communication and respect for one another's roles has been established, the team as a whole can work out solutions. For example, the therapist may be able to give in-service training to nurses in making transfers or in making better assessments and more complete documentation of the patient's progress in physical therapy. Energy freed by resolving conflicts can be directed more fully toward helping the patient and family. It is important in all settings to understand the role of the person designated as a discharge consultant. An experienced discharge consultant can particularly help to integrate the new staff member into the team, asking pertinent questions of the new therapist to facilitate discharge planning. Given an effective framework, new staff should be able to join the team without major problems. The support and shared experience both of other team members and of the therapy department ideally lead to the development of the individual therapist into an effective member of the discharge planning team.

The five steps of the discharge planning process (assessment, diagnosis, prescription, implementation, and evaluation) discussed elsewhere in this book can also be used by the physical therapist. These steps can be used in developing discharge plans or in retrospectively identifying errors. The terms "diagnosis" and "prescription" which are usually defined as physician responsibilities may be better described for physical therapists as "statement of the problem" and "creation of a plan." Utilizing these five steps in discharge planning may be most helpful for newer graduates. More-experienced therapists may already be incorporating these steps into the process.

PHYSICAL THERAPIST'S ROLE IN DISCHARGE FROM THE ACUTE HOSPITAL SETTING

The therapist's most important role may be as a consultant whose function is to (1) evaluate the patient and describe problems, (2) identify short- and long-term goals, and (3) suggest ways of achieving these goals. Patients with complex physical therapy problems requiring significant muscle reeducation and therapy programs may be referred to the therapist. The pace in an acute hospital is usually fast, the therapist probably having no more than 30 minutes to treat each patient each day. The therapist will need to set priorities and often make recommendations regarding the need for further physical therapy in another setting.

The therapist needs to communicate this information by chart documentation. The therapist may want to "flag" the chart to alert staff to read the therapy note if it is located in a separate area of the chart. The therapist should continually communicate with the person most directly responsible for coordinating with the patient his discharge plan. A concise summary of the patient's status is more valuable than several pages of evaluation. Development of evaluation guidelines may help therapists focus on important tests for specific disabilities. A form such as that shown on p. 149 is an example of an evaluative tool that could be adapted for use in many physical therapy settings.

For an orthopedic patient, accurate testing of the joint for range of motion would be indicated for the affected extremities. For the stroke patient, expanded evaluation of tone, synergy, sensation, and functional activities would be indicated. This form might also be adapted for chronic respiratory patients who are medically stable and for whom discharge is being discussed, since an evaluation of parameters other than the patient's respiratory status is also important in identifying discharge problems.

Each acute care facility will shape its multidisciplinary team to best meet its own staffing patterns. For example, one therapist might need to speak for several others when daily rounds are indicated. All therapists covering the particular unit might wish to be present when weekly rounds are held. When reporting on the patient's status, the therapist should concentrate on problems that have been identified from the assessment. An example of a useful summary follows:

PHYSICAL THERAPY: INITIAL/DISCHARGE EVALUATION

Diagnosis: __________

Social history: __________

MUSCLE STRENGTH	RANGE OF MOTION	COMMENTS
Upper extremities		
Lower extremities		

Functional activities: __________

Bed mobility: __________
Transfer: __________
Ambulation: __________
Stairs: __________
Wheelchair: __________

Other (sensation, respiratory, skin condition): __________

PROBLEMS	PT GOALS

Program: __________

Date Signature

1. Strength: patient needs increased strength in both lower extremities to ambulate safely with a walker.
2. Range of motion: I have been unable to increase the patient's hip movement in the past week. The patient will need 20° more flexion in order to safely sit and complete activities of daily living.
3. Discharge: patient is not ready for discharge. I believe that more intensive therapy would allow the patient to go home within two or three weeks.

As a result of the discussion about the patient, application may be made to a rehabilitation hospital. At this point, discharge planning at the acute hospital often ends. The patient may not even be discussed any longer except to note that he is awaiting transfer. The waiting period may last as long as several weeks, and during that time the patient may significantly improve. The physical therapist may be one of the few health professionals working with the patient during this time. The therapist needs to recognize improvements that might allow the patient to go home instead of to the rehabilitation hospital and should discuss this change with other team members. Continued involvement of a discharge planning consultant can facilitate discharge to a different destination.

For patients who have not reached their maximum potential in physical therapy in the acute hospital, a number of questions must be considered by the therapist in planning discharge:

1. Will further therapy significantly help this patient, and if not, what help and equipment will the patient need before returning home?
2. What is the patient's age, diagnosis, and medical status? (Be cautious about age, since it may be an insignificant factor and may stigmatize an older patient unnecessarily.)
3. Does the patient desire to participate in a therapy program?
4. How much is the patient able to participate?

The patient and significant other persons need to be involved in the discussion of these questions. It may not be realistic for all staff members to meet with the patient or family or both to discuss this issue. The primary person involved in coordinating discharge planning can help decide who might best meet with the patient and family. An accurate knowledge of community resources is imperative so that patients and families can realistically make decisions.

Opportunity exists for much creative thinking and planning by therapists in acute hospital settings. To improve discharge planning, the therapist, with the multidisciplinary team, should review each step and develop a framework for communication with other members so that the goal of better patient care can be met.

PHYSICAL THERAPIST'S ROLE IN DISCHARGE FROM THE REHABILITATION HOSPITAL OR UNIT

In the rehabilitation setting the patient routinely receives services from multiple disciplines, and the therapy program is usually complex and of many months' duration. The physical therapist is significantly involved in patient and family teaching, and makes recommendations for needed equiment and for home visits. Physical therapy assessment of discharge problems necessarily must be more detailed and comprehensive than in an acute care setting. An example of a form used in one rehabilitation hospital to document problems is shown on pp. 151-152. It is important that guidelines accompany these forms to help staff properly assess patients.

Communication that is ongoing, is clearly documented, and gives evidence of multidisciplinary involvement is important in developing a successful discharge plan for the complex rehabilitation patient. An example of a problem-oriented sys-

PHYSICAL THERAPY
INITIAL/DISCHARGE EVALUATION

DIAGNOSIS: 8/22 ulcer 8/24 debridement Left lower extremity R great toenail removal.
9/15 circumferential full-thickness skin graft L calf
1961 L ankle fx with pinning. History angina; thoracic kyphosis

INTRODUCTION—SOCIAL HISTORY Pt. is a delightful 71 Y.O. WF admitted to MRH 10/4/78 from MGH for medical care/wound healing. Pt. had been on bed rest following LE skin graft (as above) and was then referred to PT for progressive ambulation starting 11/3/78.

Pt. is pleasant, well motivated, and oriented. She lives alone in 7th-floor apartment in Boston with elevator. She is retired and has a variety of interests (crafts, music). Plan: to return home--probably week of 12/11.

MUSCLE STRENGTH AND RANGE OF MOTION

		STR (LEFT)	ROM (LEFT)	STR (RIGHT)	ROM (RIGHT)	COMMENTS:
SHLD.	Flexion 0-160	G–	WNL*	G–	WNL*	
	Extension 0-50	↓	↓	↓	↓	
	Abduct. 0-160	↓	↓	↓	↓	
	In. Rot. 0-70	↓	↓	↓	↓	
	Ex. Rot. 0-90	↓	↓	↓	↓	
	Sitting Pushups	↓	/////////////	↓	/////////////	
ELBOW	Flexion 0-145	G	WNL*	G	WNL*	
	Extension 0-0	↓	↓	↓	↓	
WRIST	Flexion 0-70	↓	↓	↓	↓	
	Extension 0-70	↓	↓	↓	↓	Old fx R wrist
	Pronat. 0-70	↓	↓	↓	↓	Arthritic deformities R hand
	Supin. 0-85	↓	↓	↓	↓	R handed
GRASP			COMMENTS			
HIP	St. Leg Raise	//////	WNL*	//////	WNL*	
	Flexion 0-120	G	↓	G	↓	
	Extension 0-25	↓	↓	↓	↓	
	Abduct. 0-45	↓	↓	↓	↓	
	Abduct. 0-30	↓	↓	↓	↓	
	In. Rot. 0-45	↓	↓	↓	↓	
	Ex. Rot. 0-45	↓	↓	↓	↓	
KNEE	Flexion 0-135	↓	↓	↓	↓	
	Extension 0-0			↓		
ANKLE	Dorsiflex 0-20	F+	P-20°/A-25°	↓	0-0	Has long-standing equinus
	Plantiflex	F	20-45	↓	WNL*	deformity and arthrofibrosis
	Invers. 0-35	0	0-0	↓	↓	L ankle
	Eversion 0-20	0	0-5	↓	↓	
TRUNK	Mobility	thoracic kyphosis				Old L ankle fx, 1961
	Strength	at least fair				

SENSATION
c/o numbness/tingling of hands--intermittent
appears intact all extremities to lt. touch, proprioception, pinprick.

RESPIRATORY
Nonremarkable; endurance is good.

SKIN CONDITION LLE s/p FTSG to calf area (circumferential area is pink, covered with Vaseline gauze and dressings). Is allowed FWB. R thigh donor site--pink, well healed. LLE is edematous below the knee. Bony enlargement at lateral malleolus 2° to old fx.

*Within normal limits.

Continued.

PHYSICAL THERAPY: INITIAL/DISCHARGE EVALUATION—CONT'D

FUNCTIONAL ACTIVITIES

	UNABLE	ASST.	SUP.	IND.	COMMENTS
ROLLING				X	
SUPINE TO SIT				X	
SIT TO STAND				XX	
W/C TRANSFERS				X	
W/C MOBILITY				X	
STAIRS				X	Uses walker and railing
SITTING BALANCE				X	Normal
STANDING BALANCE				X	Good

GAIT (Asst. required, devices, deviations, endurances, etc.)

Ambulates independently on level and uneven surfaces with walker
Endurance is 300 ft.

(Have attempted to progress to hemiwalker or quadcane, however this causes increased pain L ankle and antalgic gait)

OTHER (Coordination, special tests, etc.)

PROBLEMS	P.T. GOALS
1. Pain & stiffness L ankle	1. Decrease pain, increase mobility Pt. performs own active LE exercises
2. LLE minimally edematous with healing skin graft	2. Decrease edema
3. Ambulation requires walker	3. Eventually progress to lesser assistive device. (Post discharge will ask VNA PT to follow up)

PROGRAM

RPT will follow until D/C home anticipated wk of 12/11.
Home visit does not seem necessary at this time.

Equipment--Pt. has own walker and raised toilet seat at home.

L.H., RPT — Signature

12/4/78 — Date

PHYSICAL THERAPY FLOWCHART

Date: 3/20 PROBLEMS	*Date:* 3/22 Therapist: S. Jones, RPT	*Date:* 3/29 Therapist: S. Jones, RPT	*Date:* Therapist:	*Date:* Therapist:	*Date:* 3/22 PT goals
1 Decreased L knee flexion passively to 90° actively to 110°	Actively and passively to 110°	Actively and passively to 110°			Knee flexion to 135°
2 Decreased quadriceps strength	Maximum 2 lb	Maximum 6 lb			Ability to lift 20 lb x 30 repetitions
3 Ambulation: requiring 2 crutches	2 crutches	2 crutches			Independent without devices

Primary diagnoses: s/p (L) medial meniscectomy

Related problems: None

FUNCTIONAL EVALUATION FORM

Multidisciplinary evaluation of functional capabilities for patients discharged home

Patient's name:______________ Date started:______________

Disposition: home--alone during day, family present at night

	SIGNATURE OF CARE GIVER WHO EVALUATES PROBLEM
Areas to be evaluated	
1. Independence and safety in activities of daily living	J. Jones, OT
2. Knowledge of medications	S. Doppelt, RN
3. Independence and safety in kitchen	J. Jones, OT
Date completed:______________	
Results of evaluation	
1. Independent in activities of daily living	J. Jones, OT
2. Unable to safely administer own medications	S. Doppelt, RN
3. Unsafe in kitchen area; requires constant supervision and assistance for planning	J. Jones, OT
4.	
5.	
6.	

Recommendations: Family will need assistance for medication administration during day and possibly homemaker to assist with midday meal.

S. Doppelt, RN; J. Jones, OT

tem of therapy documentation that other disciplines may find useful is shown in the flowchart on p. 153.

An excellent means of determining potential discharge problems is to simulate a home setting in the hospital and place the patient in the setting (usually for one week). A multidisciplinary team might implement this program for a week prior to anticipated discharge. A patient who is on this program is evaluated on his ability to perform the morning and evening self-care, transfers, ambulatory or wheelchair activities, toileting, bathing, some meal planning and preparation, and light household tasks. Medication and dietary instruction are provided, and recommendations are made at the completion of the program. Examples of a few problem areas to be evaluated and the results of evaluation are shown in the functional evaluation form shown above.

The success of the program depends on cooperation among all health care givers. In addition, a visit to the patient's home prior to discharge can help the team discover architectural barriers and determine the need for adaptive equipment, home services, and further training before the patient is ready to return home. A form that might be utilized to assess discharge problems on home visits is shown on pp. 155-156. Occupational and physical therapists are encouraged to make home visits and to complete the form as a team.

These tools can help the staff focus on the ultimate goal of a well-timed, smooth discharge to the optimum setting for a patient. The more objective the physical therapist is in assessing problems and creating clear plans, the easier the implementation of those plans.

HOME VISIT EVALUATION FORM

Method of locomotion (i.e., Wheelchair): ____________
Type of dwelling: apartment ____ home ____
Patient will be living: Completely alone ____ Alone part of the day ____ Rarely/never alone ____

Key: U = Unable
A = Assistance required
I = Independent (safely and effectively)
NA = Not applicable

	U	A	I	NA	COMMENTS AND RECOMMENDATIONS
1. *Describe patient's ability to negotiate*					
a. Elevators					
b. Stairs					
c. Ramps					
d. Thresholds					
e. Carpet and scatter rugs					
f. Through doorways					
g. Other obstacles (specify)					
2. *Bathroom*					
a. Ability to get to bathroom					
b. Ability to maneuver through room					
c. Ability to transfer on and off toilet					
d. Ability to transfer in and out of tub					
e. Ability to reach sink and faucet					
f. Ability to reach medicine cabinet					
3. *Kitchen*					
a. Ability to maneuver through room					
b. Ability to use table and chair					
c. Ability to reach shelves and cabinets					
d. Ability to transfer items within kitchen (e.g., dishes, pots)					
e. Ability to use utilities (e.g., refrigerator, stove, sink)					
4. *Bedroom*					
a. Ability to maneuver through room					
b. Ability to transfer in and out of bed					
c. Ability to reach necessary items (phone)					
d. Ability to use closets and drawers					
5. *Living room*					
a. Ability to maneuver through room					
b. Ability to transfer on and off chairs, couch					
c. Ability to manage TV, radio, phone					

Continued.

HOME VISIT EVALUATION FORM—CONT'D

	YES	NO	COMMENTS AND RECOMMENDATIONS
6. *Miscellaneous*			
a. Will patient be managing own laundry? If so, how?			
b. Will patient be doing all or part of cleaning? If not, who will?			
c. Will patient do own shopping? If not, who will?			
d. Are appropriate emergency numbers near phone?			
e. Can patient escape from home safely?			
f. Can family or friends assist patient safely?			

7. *Summary of recommendations:* With the above recommendations, will this be a safe discharge home? If not, why? ____________________

____

____

____

Date: ____________________ Signature: ____________________

Regular patient care conferences or team conferences are vital in the discharge planning process. If the patient is not present at these meetings, it is useful to designate a member of the team to summarize the team conference for the patient. On some rehabilitation units an initial team presentation includes patients in discussion of goals and expectations. This approach is time consuming but useful in encouraging patient involvement. Patients should be encouraged to discuss their progress on a regular basis with the therapist.

A comprehensive discharge treatment plan is often a necessity in the rehabilitation setting. The patient may have lifelong physical therapy needs (daily stretching and other exercises, splinting, or positioning). The patient will probably be discharged to a permanent setting and may require services from many agencies. When the physical therapist in the referring hospital completes, copies, and forwards a discharge evaluation form such as that shown on pp. 151-152, comprehensive and complete information is provided.

Evaluation of the effectiveness of discharge planning is a challenge for rehabilitation hospitals. Patients often return to a primary clinic for medical and other care. If distance permits, some rehabilitation hospitals have patients return for follow-up visits, providing staff with feedback on the success of the discharge plan. Follow-up can be particularly important in complex rehabilitation problems, such as spinal cord injuries or amputations, for which specialized care must be given. When a patient returns to one of the various medical clinics (e. g., orthopedic, vascular, renal, or medical), often no one comprehensively looks at the patient's functional status. A multidisciplinary primary care team utilizing a therapist as a consultant could be available to evaluate the patient's status and the success of rehabilitation efforts.

PHYSICAL THERAPIST'S ROLE IN DISCHARGE FROM AMBULATORY CARE

In ambulatory care settings, such as a visiting nurse service, private practice, a neighborhood health center, or an outpatient department of a hospital, the discharge "team" is often limited to the referring physician and the physical therapist. Most communication between the physician and therapist may be conducted by telephone or letter. The therapist, physician, and patient need to agree on goals. This agreement can allow the therapist and patient to work out a program over a reasonable time period (e.g., therapy three times per week until range of motion is normal, then once weekly until the patient is ready to progress to a home program consisting of strengthening exercises). Ambulatory patients have jobs and other commitments besides physical therapy. Thus, efficiency of treatment plans and programs is particularly important. Sharing problems and goal-oriented documentation with the patient can help clarify gains that are being made. A flowchart such as that shown on p. 153 can be an efficient means of documenting patient progress.

Discharge planning for the patient who fully recovers from an injury or problem is relatively easy. Some patients referred for therapy, however, do not fully recover. Deciding when to discharge these patients can become difficult, particularly in view of the problems in arranging meetings with the physician. A problem-oriented summary that includes goals reached and recommendations made can be sent with the patient to the physician to provide the information necessary for discharge of the patient. Patients will be less likely to feel abandoned, particularly when only partial recovery of function is possible, if the therapist and physician agree on goals and a time framework for reaching these goals at the time the patient begins therapy.

PHYSICAL THERAPIST'S ROLE IN DISCHARGE FROM THE NURSING HOME

Depending on licensure, the nursing home may be expected to provide only minimum physical therapy services. Often the therapist may be utilized as a consultant, and therapy and nursing aides are responsible for treatment. As a consultant, the therapist might begin by systematically evaluating *all* patients, not just those referred for physical therapy. An evaluation form similar to that shown on p. 149 could be developed and used in designing programs for patients. Patients, nursing home staff, and family members need to be included in helping the patient maintain independence or achieve greater independence. (For example, someone with carpentry skills might construct a board that can be placed under the patient's wheelchair to improve balance.) Some patients are able to make sufficient improvement so that discharge from the nursing home can be considered. Careful physical therapy assessment, program planning, and reassessment of gains are necessary before such a discharge is initiated.

PHYSICAL THERAPIST'S ROLE IN EVALUATION OF THE DISCHARGE PLANNING PROCESS

Improving discharge planning requires accurate information about how well or how poorly patients have done after discharge. Time spent by physical therapists in obtaining this information can be costly and is generally not reimbursable. Some ways in which therapists can participate in evaluation of discharges include the following:

1. Suggesting audit topics (e.g., follow-up of amputees from a facility) or elements of a multidisciplinary audit (e.g., whether patients are able to ambulate independently on discharge, or are able to don prostheses independently). Hospital quality assurance committees are interested in such audits.
2. Participating in clinics (e.g., neurology, arthritis, or pulmonary). A therapist there would reassess the patient's status and change home programs accordingly.
3. Developing a system of peer review. Standards should include clear documentation from admission to discharge. The American Physical Therapy Association has resource material to help in developing peer review systems.
4. Sharing problems and successes in discharge planning with therapists from other hospitals.

SUMMARY

The physical therapist plays a specific role on the multidisciplinary team responsible for planning discharge from the acute hospital, rehabilitation facility, nursing home, or outpatient setting. Based on objective evaluation of a patient's functioning, the therapist can develop guidelines for more effective discharge planning. This chapter offers a framework for understanding the process of discharge planning from the point of view of the physical therapist.

ACKNOWLEDGMENT

The author is grateful to the Massachusetts Rehabilitation Hospital for use of its forms as examples.

REFERENCE

1. American Physical Therapy Association: Policy log, abridged version, Washington, D.C., Jan., 1978, the Association, p. 70.

ADDITIONAL READINGS

American Physical Therapy Association: Competencies in physical therapy: an analysis of practice, San Diego, 1977, Courseware.

Brody, E. M.: Long-term care of older people, New York, 1977, Human Sciences Press.

Brook, R. H., Appel, F. A., Avery, C., and others: Effectiveness of inpatient follow-up care, N. Engl. J. Med. **285**:1509-1514, 1971.

Commission on Accreditation of Rehabilitation Facilities: Standards manual for rehabilitation facilities, Chicago, 1978, the Commission.

Department of Health, Education, and Welfare: Federal health insurance for the aged and disabled, Washington, D.C., 1975, Federal Register.

Department of Public Health, Commonwealth of Massachusetts: Licensure rules and regulations for hospitals in Massachusetts, Boston, 1971, the Department.

Joint Commission of Accreditation of Hospitals: Accreditation manual for hospitals, Chicago, 1971, the Commission.

Schuman, J. E., and Willard, H. N.: Role of the acute hospital team in planning discharge of the chronically ill, Geriatrics **31**:63-67, 1976.

Schuman, J. E., Ostfeld, A. M., and Willard, H. N.: Discharge planning in an acute hospital, Arch. Phys. Med. Rehabil. **57**:343-347, 1976.

Wise, H., et al.: Making health teams work, Cambridge, Mass., 1974, Ballinger Publishing Co.

CHAPTER 13

Discharge planning: an occupational therapist's perspective

MICHAEL J. STEINHAUER

The occupational therapist uses a variety of activities to return a client to the highest possible level of independence in his physical, mental, social, recreational, vocational, and economic life. When the acute phase of illness has passed, the occupational therapist utilizes a program of rehabilitation training and simulated environments to gain from the client desired physical and mental responses. The client is then assessed from a functional viewpoint; the goal is to help the individual return to prehospitalization activities when possible. Occupational therapy may be used with all diagnostic groups of clients in a variety of settings. The occupational therapist works with the whole person, concentrating on the quality of the client's life while considering human sciences, the art of selected activity, and specific precautions related to the client's disability. To accomplish these tasks, the occupational therapist works closely with the health care team to educate other disciplines in understanding the unique perspective and training of the profession.

In the rehabilitation and discharge planning process, it is crucial to communicate with other team members and be familiar with their professional philosophies and techniques. The process of defining and coordinating roles minimizes the possibility that the needs of the client will be threatened by professional ego or territorial feelings. In my experience the team members on any specified unit rarely changed, and if they did change, a rotating occupational therapist was assigned who had previously worked with the same team members. This practice led to increased communication and understanding of each professional's strengths and weaknesses; thus the treatment goals could be apportioned among the team members, and consistency of approach could be ensured. The discharge planning process is enhanced further by the appointment of a team leader or coordinator assigned to call and conduct meetings, assess the client's total program, and mediate professionally threatening circumstances. The leader is most often an individual who has worked closely with all disciplines and who has input into the client's program around the clock. Nursing staff most adequately meet these criteria. The client is then not treated in one clinic for an arm and in another for a leg; he is viewed as a whole person. Clients perceive this multidisciplinary communication during the rehabilitation process, and it influences their understanding of, response to, and cooperation with the program. The therapist relies on this understanding to demonstrate that rehabilitation is a philosophy, and not only a physical or psychiatric treatment technique.

The intent of this chapter is to highlight an occupational therapist's perspective in discharge planning and to illustrate guidelines. Occupational therapists are found in a variety of settings. However, the format for this chapter was chosen to address the adult client's physical or emotional disability, and to consider two possible settings to which a client may return or be transferred after discharge: the community or the extended care facility.

GUIDING CONSIDERATIONS IN THE DISCHARGE PLANNING PROCESS

There are four considerations that guide the occupational therapist in the process of discharge planning. The following material addresses these considerations and highlights some ideas that may be utilized in conjunction with each consideration. The four considerations are client participation, the expertise of the multidisciplinary team, the use of community resources, and the influence of the family or significant other persons (Fig. 13-1).

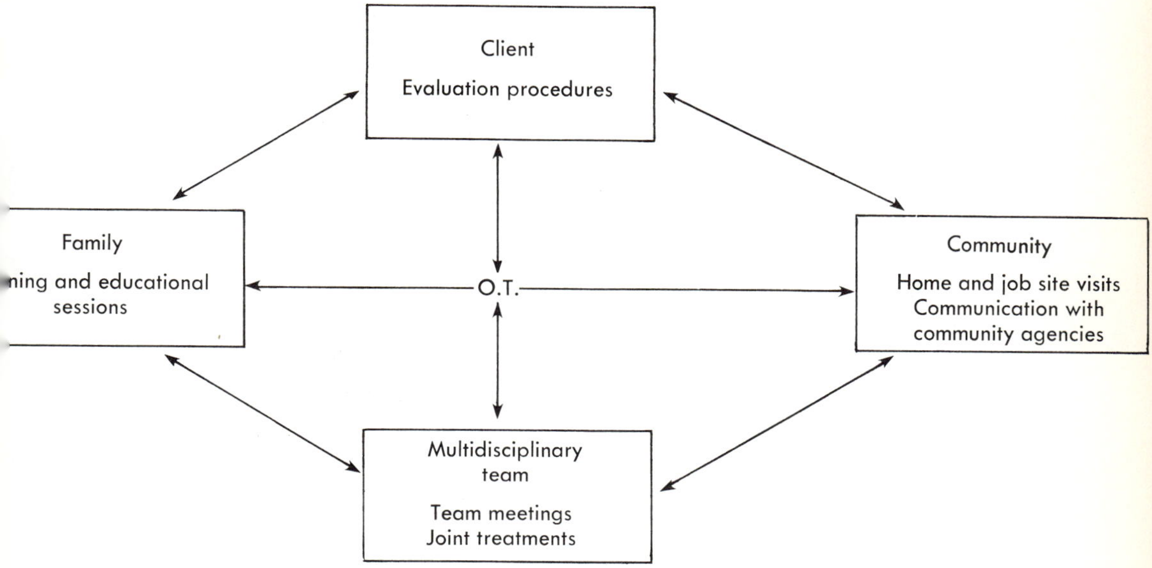

Fig. 13-1. Guiding considerations in the discharge planning process.

Client participation

The therapist is constantly monitoring the client's response to treatment, including the client's concept of self, psychological adjustment to the disability, and level of learning ability. The therapist also should observe the client's commitment to and involvement in the program. Frequent interviews will assist the occupational therapist in determining the client's response to treatment and will provide opportunities for reassessment. In long-term rehabilitation settings, clients and therapists develop a close relationship. Life-styles and dreams are shared, information is exchanged, and a vital sense of partnership is established. When communication skills and the therapeutic relationship are used, the client can be encouraged to attain the desired goal. Yet, although the therapist evaluates the effectiveness of treatment and documents this process, occupational therapy does not judge the life-style that a client had prior to admittance to the institution. For example, the client who, before hospitalization, bathed once a week may be encouraged to do so more often for a variety of hygienic reasons, but the goals of treatment are not intended to alter that specific behavior. They are intended to retrain the client to accomplish the task only, but in the final analysis the client chooses his own life-style, and nobody else's. Assuming that clients are able to make decisions for themselves without harming others, it is essential that they maintain these individual rights to life-style.

Expertise of the multidisciplinary team

Another guiding factor in the discharge planning process is the occupational therapist's level of communication with other team members and his ability to interpret their expertise. The client's prognosis, the medical contraindications to postdischarge activities, and the effects of medications are all important considerations. Team meetings provide a good mechanism for communication among health care professionals. Meetings that are structured to encourage questions and pose concerns can lead to a healthy exchange of information and ideas. Gaining both insight into team strengths and an understanding of the need to obtain certain services outside the institution can be discussed. To participate in the process, the client also may attend some meetings. This educational experience will allow the client to see at first hand the professional's perspective and the team's decision-making process.

Use of community resources

Discharge planning also necessitates an awareness of the culture and economic structure of the community in which the client lives. Ethnic pride, availability of public or private funds, housing, recreational centers, and job opportunities are important considerations in planning for discharge. *A plan for discharge is only as good as the evaluation of the client and his environment*. Home and community visits are useful. Evaluating the place of employment and recreational facilities should be included in the assessment procedure. Information concerning architec-

CLIENT QUESTIONNAIRE
ON HOME ENVIRONMENT

Directions: You can assist us by completing the following questionnaire. This information will help us to plan the rehabilitation program for

______________________.
(Patient's name)

I. *Preliminary family information*
   A. Number of people living in home or nearby (please specify): ________
   B. Ages of people living in home: ____, ____, ____, ____, ____, ____
   C. Person who would be primarily responsible for home care (if needed): ________
      1. Is this person in good general health? ________
      2. Will this person be living in the home? ________
      3. Does this person work? ________
      4. Can the responsible person come to the hospital in a weekday between 8:00 A.M. and 4:00 P.M. for instruction in home care program? Yes____ No ____

II. *Client social and recreational activities*
   Please list a few activities the client enjoyed while living at home. Include daily schedule.

III. *Evaluation of architectural/structural status*
   A. Physical layout
      1. Apartment ____ 1-family house ____ 2-family house ____
      2. No. of floors: ____ Elevator ____ Walk-up ____
      3. Carpeting: Wall-to-wall Scatter
   B. Entrance
      1. Location of most often used and accessible--front, side, or back: ________
      2. No. of steps: ________
      3. Width of door: ________
      4. Railing: ________ Both sides? ________
      5. Floor covering: ________
   C. Family rooms
      1. Living room size and accessibility (chairs): ________
      2. Dining room (chairs): ________
      3. Den (if any): ________
      4. Other: ________
      5. Floor covering: ________
   D. Bathroom
      1. Toilet height and accessibility (with wheelchair or ambulatory device): ________
      2. Location (by floor[s]): ________
      3. Width of door: ________
      4. Width of room and accessibility: ________
      5. Tub information (height, type): ________
      6. Shower information (type, etc.): ________
      7. Wall construction (wood, tile): ________
      8. Fixtures (easily usable?): ________
      9. Floor covering: ________

Continued.

tural barriers, the employer-client relationship, and on-site mobility factors (e.g., use of walkers, wheelchairs, and bathroom assistive devices) can all be incorporated into the treatment plan. Simulated work and recreational situations can be practiced in the clinic. Space accessibility, energy conservation techniques, adaptive equipment, and work simplication training are all considered when treatments oriented toward returning the client to the community are planned.

Influence of the family or significant others

Although most guiding considerations will center around the client directly, the therapist may be able to include the influence and assistance of the family and of significant other person such as clergy and friends. Understanding the dynamics of

CLIENT QUESTIONNAIRE ON HOME ENVIRONMENT—CONT'D

E. Kitchen
1. Accessibility (with wheelchair or ambulatory device?): ______
2. Cabinet accessibility: ______
3. Fixtures (usable?): ______
4. Rough diagram of major appliances and furniture (e.g., stove, refrigerator, table): ______

F. Bedroom
1. Accessibility (with wheelchair or ambulatory device?): ______
2. Height of bed: ______
3. Closet and bureau accessibility: ______
4. Floor covering: ______

FLOOR PLAN

Signature of person completing form: ______

Date: ______

Relationship: ______

these interpersonal relationships before and during the client's hospitalization will provide valuable information if these persons will be assisting the client in achieving the desired goals. For example, the handicapped ex-athlete can still fill a needed role on the football team by encouraging and supporting fellow team members. The client who has been driven to succeed in therapy by his teammates may return to the field as the coach's assistant, the timekeeper, a talent scout, or the like. The significant others not only may greatly influence the client by giving understanding and support but also may themselves be encouraged, through their participation, to appropriately interpret the illness. It is helpful to use a client-and-home questionnaire, completed by a family member, to provide information about the client's home and community environment. This information, which should be requested soon after admission facilitates family involvement in the program. For a sample questionnaire, see pp. 163-164.

THE CLIENT

Although frames of reference and theoretical models may differ from clinic to clinic and from therapist to therapist, every occupational therapist considers similar client assessment areas when planning for discharge. Some of these areas include psychological adjustment, activities of daily living skills, and social and recreational needs. In some areas, factors may vary according to whether the client has a physical or a mental disability.

The client with a physical disability

Psychological adjustment and transitional support. Occupational therapists directly explore the psychological makeup of a client prior to discharge so that acceptability and effectiveness of the discharge plan can be evaluated. A social worker, psychiatrist, or other health care professional may be asked to assist in determining emotional difficulties arising from the client's response to his disability. Some examples of emotional difficulty include negative feelings toward persons who react awkwardly toward a handicapped person, sexual identity fears, and fear of rejection. Family members' responses are also noted, and counseling of both family and client is often begun simultaneously. The family members must make their own adjustment to the client's situation, and their ability to do so will influence the client.

If the client is to be discharged to an extended care facility, the therapist will continue to provide support so that transition is not seen as a threatening or failing experience. Instead, the client is encouraged to view the placement as an opportunity to continue to work on the rehabilitation goals still to be achieved. The importance of succinct referral writing is stressed here, because it is important to maintain a consistent approach and to establish communication between therapists.

Role of the family. The success or failure of a rehabilitation or discharge plan may depend on the reaction and adjustment ability of the family or significant others. The stability of the client's self-concept is often maintained within his interpersonal relationships. This self-concept may therefore be either threatened or enhanced, as the client accepts the challenge of rehabilitation and discharge, by negative or positive family attitudes. The occupational therapist can structure treatments to encourage or establish a positive attitude in the family through several mechanisms. One such mechanism is education. Active learning-and-doing sessions can change a devastating picture of illness into a manageable responsibility. Any family member or significant other can participate—even the youngest member who has an influence on the client. These family teaching sessions can begin with a basic understanding of function and pathology relevant to the client's illness. Meetings may also stress the principles of therapeutically graded activities and compensatory techniques such as utilizing assistive devices. A good exercise for family members may be to have participants place themselves in the role of the client, with similar limitations and skills. This technique may help the participants "feel" more realistically the client's reality. Educational sessions may also help the family conquer the fear and embarrassment of actually touching the client's affected area. With these experiences the client and family will gain a greater sense of security with the rehabilitation program and then in turn will assist the therapist in laying the groundwork for a smooth transition at discharge.

The following situation illustrates the family's application of these educational sessions at home. An elderly woman has suffered a stroke affecting her right side. It has been determined that the family will be responsible to care for the client's personal hygiene, particularly in assisting with transfers into the tub at home. After education the family members are more knowledgeable and comfortable in handling the affected limbs and understand the difficulties of motion, sensation, and communication that the client experiences. Educational sessions have also enabled the family to work with assistive devices such as grab bars and tub seats. It is important for the client to perceive the ease and confidence that family members have attained. Family members may, however, tend to shy away from these educational sessions if they are overconfident of their ability to adjust. However, these sessions can often bring previously unidentified feelings to the surface and provide an atmosphere in which they may be worked out—but not at the client's expense.

Social and recreational needs. The onset of a disability does not connote the cessation of a needed balance between work and play. The client who suffers from a disabling condition will undoubtedly express concern for returning to a life that contains some social or recreational time. After a comprehensive evaluation of a client's interests and hobbies, the therapist should indicate to the client the need to redefine the term "play" in the light of a new set of abilities and limitations. As is often the case, educating the client and providing him with an assistive device(s) will place many goals within reach. For example, a card shuffler and automatic dealer may take the place of a client's arthritic hands at the Wednesday night bridge game.

Other skills, such as sexual functioning and social acceptability, are not just a matter of appropriate client-equipment compatibility. The therapist needs to rely on the counseling services of such professionals as social workers and recreation therapists. In addition, extended teaching sessions for close friends will give the client and all significant others an opportunity to explore feelings and present solutions in a structured setting.

Assistive devices: prescription and utilization. Assistive devices are certainly one of the main responsibilities of the occupational therapist. He should know what devices are available, which devices to prescribe for a particular client, how to fabricate various devices, and how to provide instruction in their use. When discharge of a client who has a physical handicap is planned, these devices may be the answer to many problems that cause client and family despair and directly affect the rehabilitation potential of the client.

There are several points that should be highlighted. First, the occupational

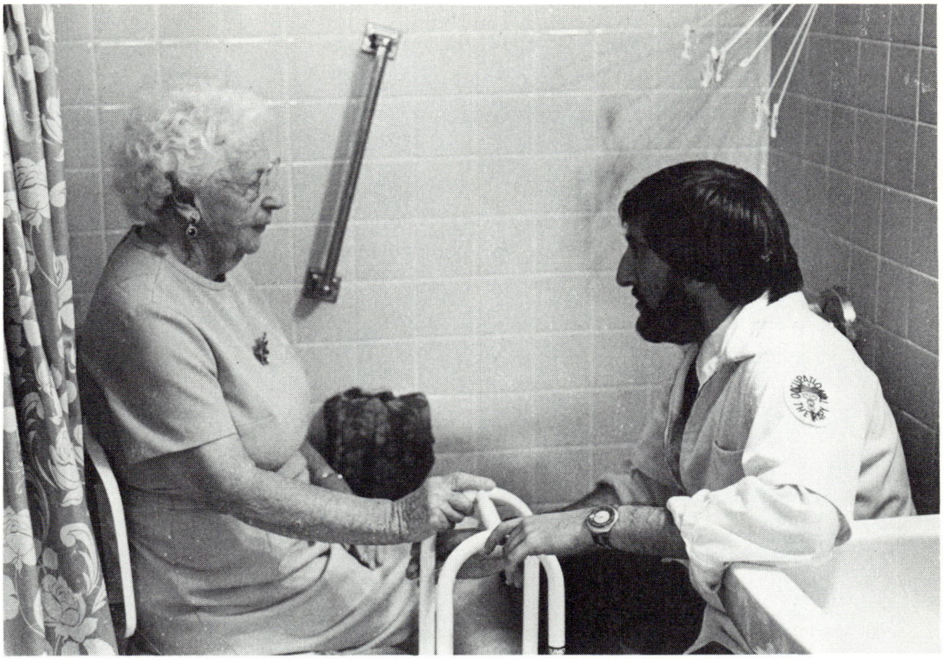

Fig. 13-2. Occupational therapist reviewing transfer procedures with client during home evaluation. Assistive devices have been borrowed from occupational therapy clinic to ensure appropriate equipment orders prior to discharge. (Courtesy Senior Home Care Services, Boston, and Peter Kennedy.)

therapist should make an accurate diagnosis of the client's skills, taking into account the contraindications of certain motions and deficits of the muscular and nervous systems. Second, the client should be available to practice the use of devices while an inpatient, to ensure that equipment orders are appropriate and timely. It is advised that therapists attempt to acquaint themselves with the local medical supplier, who can be a valuable source of information and service. Third, the cost of an item is to be considered. Overburdening the family or third-party payers with catalog costs for equipment may be unnecessary. Explore the potential for homemade devices if possible. Finally, the client's acceptance of a device is important to ensure that the skills and cooperation are utilized to the fullest. The client may need to be encouraged to accept new devices to achieve goals. In addition, the client needs to understand that the recommendations for equipment are for *self-help* purposes and that a piece of equipment is not to be viewed as an uncontrolled object that dictates self-worth.

Self-help devices may hold the key to avoiding the often embarrassing and self-degrading experience of having to rely on others to achieve a task. The therapist should include the family members in the securing of devices, however, by educating them on the methods of ordering additional parts from the medical supply companies and on the care and maintenance of equipment.

Activities of daily living and mobility. With the increase of rehabilitation techniques, occupational therapy has expanded its role and now has the capacity to train disabled persons to increase their skills in all areas. Activites of daily living (ADL), no longer just the criteria of self-care management, may include transportation, communication, hand activities as they relate to social and vocational skills, and all homemaking skills. Driver training is also a part of occupational therapy. Therapists train clients in transfer abilities, perceptual-motor skills, and organization and concentration skills. Each client is evaluated as needing either specialized instruction and guidance or assistive devices.

Mobility skills relate directly to a client's performance level and the plan for discharge. Expectations and treatment plans for ambulatory clients are different from those for wheelchair-bound clients or for clients who will use a wheelchair to accomplish a task. In ADL and mobility training sessions, where wheelchair use will affect transportation needs and homemaking and vocational skills, therapists will review the following exercises: reaching elevator buttons, maneuvering up ramps, negotiating through narrow doorways and over curbs, and preparing meals with long-handled devices. When the client is ambulatory (with or without assistive devices for stability), the therapist will teach accommodation to stairs and curbs and will review the use of some equipment for these more mobile clients. Seat canes, walker aprons, and baskets for carrying items are most commonly used.

In most ADL and mobility training sessions a complete work-motion analysis is done, and an attempt may be made to closely simulate the work and home environments. The specific activities required are broken down to their simplest form and then advanced in complexity while the client is working with the necessary equipment. For self-care skills the use of a tub seat, raised toilet seat, sliding boards, and grab bars may be rehearsed in the hospital, and then these devices may be incorporated into the architectural features of the home, job site, or extended care facility. In homemaker training, the use of an adapted kitchen in the occupational therapy clinic is recommeded to prepare the client to work independently and safely. This environment will closely simulate the home kitchen after architectural changes have been made and equipment recommendations followed. Work efficiency, safety, and energy conservation are stressed.

When the client's performance is analyzed in terms of the relative simplicity or complexity of various activites, all skills that could be used in the development of self-care and other ADL skills are initially assessed. Examples of these beginning skills are bed mobility (i.e., turning, rising, and sitting in bed), sitting or standing balance and tolerance, and ability to perform transfers. Proper application of these skills to the more complex functional skills of eating, grooming, maintaining oral hygiene, bathing, and dressing is made. For example, as a client's standing tolerance and balance increases, the ability to participate in standing showers increases. If the client can stand only long enough for a stand-pivot transfer, however, then a bath seat is recommended for use in the shower. Grab bars and safety rails may be used also, depending on the type of environment the client will enter after discharge and his need for added stability.

It may not be necessary for the occupational therapist to train a client in each self-care skill. Members of the support system, particularly home health aides, may be responsible for assisting the client in a specific activity. Family members may also assist with some activities when mechanical or assistive devices are not sufficient. Certainly clients are encouraged to do as much for themselves as possible, but when safety is threatened, support services are good compensatory mechanisms. The earlier support services are indicated as being needed to assist the client, the sooner training can begin.

Perceptual skills, concentration, and decision making. The occupational therapist is beginning to study the client's visual perceptual fields for the purpose of incorporating information regarding deficits into an appropriate discharge plan. Studies are also being made to determine the effects of mental illness on perceptual field function. Figure ground, spatial relations, depth perception, and other perceptual skills are noted in the description of the client's abilities. The client's cognitive skills, such as abstract reasoning or mathematical ability, will dictate the appropriateness of a plan for employment. Several of the evaluation techniques practiced in the occupational therapy clinic will test the client's ability to perform simple to complex tasks. For example, the client's performance in working with crafts may be analyzed, or a standardized perceptual evaluation may be made. If the client is to be discharged to a home or sheltered workshop situation or is to be referred to a prevocational training program, the client's work will probably be task oriented and should not be overstimulating perceptually or cognitively. Ability to follow directions, appropriateness of frustration responses, and decision-making and problem-solving skills are also noted. Simulation exercises, group feedback sessions, and assertiveness training may be included in the course of treatment for clients having both physical and emotional difficulties.

Therapeutic exercise after discharge. Every client should understand the consequences of not consistently practicing the regimen of exercises designed to lead to the highest level of wellness. The client's understanding, cooperation, and trust, as well as his ability to incorpoate these exercises into daily life patterns are crucial. The therapist assists in this effort by designing simple exercises and then illustrating them. Teaching may be complemented by handout sheets or written instruction, preferably accompanied by pictures or diagrams. It is important that the client and all members of the support systems be aware of bodily signs and symptoms of fatigue, such as shortness of breath, profuse sweating, and increased pulse. Members of the multidisciplinary team can greatly assist in this effort by adding their own expertise. For example, the nutritionist may discuss diet, or the physical therapist may provide input on the prescribed exercises. Instructions for these exercises should be forwarded to the agencies and individuals who will work with the client, such as the visiting nurse association, extended care facilities, private duty nurses, and all family members or significant others.

The client with an emotional disability

Some discharge considerations for clients with an emotional disability are similar to those for clients who have a physical disability. Clients with an emotional disability need to work toward developing more *basic* living skills and responsibilities that must be faced after discharge. In the mental health field, occupational therapists concentrate on providing a level of care that focuses on preventing fixation and regression as well as loss of function and self-esteem.

Concept of self and other ego functions. In the discharge planning process the client's self-esteem, body image, and related functional ability will influence the final decisions on extended care placement, level of independent living, and follow-up requirements. The client with poor self-esteem will have difficulty finding supportiveness and acceptance in the working and social worlds. An appropriate discharge plan considers the client's realistic perception of his own assets and limitations, as well as his interest orientation, need for reward, and ability to accept failure. Many projective techniques highlight objects and actions that may help to bring subconscious feelings to the surface. In using these techniques, the occupational therapist reviews the client's organization, strength, symbolism, resistiveness, and other responses through art or sentence completion exercises. After these points are assessed, success-oriented treatment, with an emphasis on performance, is begun by using structured tasks to reach a desired goal. Self-discovery games and values clarification exercises will help the client to reach some goals. Discharge-oriented treatment is aimed at providing situations and experiences that produce minimum stress for the client. Examples of a stress-producing experience include failure to perform a task, and rejection. If progress is made in the client's ability to accept some of these stresses, more-challenging experiences may be attempted. The therapist comprehensively evaluates each work or play situation a client may enter after discharge to determine the appropriateness of the client's involvement. Individual or group treatment sessions that simulate environments outside the institution may be recommended. These exercises work toward achieving a client's higher self-image and developing necessary coping mechanisms.

Communication level. The nature and manner of a client's ability to communicate his own thoughts and feelings are subjects of concern for occupational therapists planning discharge care. Verbal and nonverbal communication may be indicative of stress-producing situations. Assertiveness training, role playing, and other simulation activities (e.g., a recreation group), will assist the client in preparing to cope with the pressures of economic and social demands. Cooperation, team organization, group feelings, and spontaneous expression are monitored and applied to the discharge plan.

Activities of daily living and other self-care skills. Many of the same considerations regarding ADL and other self-care skills that were mentioned earlier, in the discussion of clients with a physical disability, are relevant when discharge from a mental health setting is planned. Although assistive devices are not utilized as often with clients who have emotional difficulties, the principles of a healthy self-esteem and body image are reflected through proper appearance and self-management. They in turn contribute to the client's acceptance into the working and social worlds. Proper appearance is often the job interviewer's criterion for judging the desirability of an applicant with a mental health history. The occupational therapist uses simulated or actual environments to monitor the client's ability to handle money, appropriately interpret time, care for his surroundings, and use public transportation. A good way to monitor ADL skills while planning for discharge is to create a community exploration group. This group of clients, led by the occupational therapist explores the community by means of field trips and real-life experiences. These activities promote a greater understanding and awareness of community facilities, such as social clubs and transportation systems, and help to develop individual interests of clients.

Influence and assistance of family. As noted earlier, involvement of family members or significant others can play a key role in the successful implementation of discharge plans. Family meetings and client-family discussion sessions are recommended. If stress-producing situations are present, the family may affect the client in such a way as to inhibit performance in some areas. The final discharge plan rests with attempts to resolve family problems as they relate to the client. The client should be assured that the family will cooperate to meet discharge goals.

DISCHARGE SETTINGS

Discharge to home or community

Architectural barriers and environmental adaptations. It is useless to train a client to use assistive devices in functional activities, only to have him return to a home that is a structural barrier to maximum performance. Developing an objective tool for evaluating home and community environments is recommended. Through the use of adaptive equipment, structural changes, and human support systems, each home or job site can become a place where the client can achieve maximum safe independence. (Examples of occupational therapy assessment forms may be seen on pp. 172-175. The restaurant accessibility form may be kept on file in the clinic for further reference by other therapists and clients.)

In addition to the therapist's assessment, clients and families need to be taught some of the criteria used to evaluate recreational, social, and vocational environments.

Family education and support. Family members and significant others are called on to participate in learning to assist in making transfers; to care for and use assistive devices, to monitor the client's signs and symptoms of fatigue, and to use the

OCCUPATIONAL THERAPY HOME
ASSESSMENT FORM

I. *Physical aspects of home*
  A. General layout
    1. Apartment_____ 1-family home_____ 2-family home_____
    2. No. of floors:_____ Elevator_____ Walk-up_____
    3. If possible, please sketch floor plan on attached page.
  B. Entrances
    1. Main entrance
      a. Number of steps:_____
      b. Width of door:_____ inches
      c. Is there a railing? Yes_____ No_____
      d. Is railing on: Right side_____ Left side_____ Both sides_____
      e. Are stairs: Circular_____ Straight_____
    2. Rear entrance
      a. Number of steps:_____
      b. Is there a railing? Yes_____ No_____
      c. Is railing on: Right side_____ Left side_____ Both sides_____
      d. Are stairs: Circular_____ Straight_____
    3. Which entrance is most commonly used?
  C. Utilities
    1. Heat? Yes_____ No_____ What type?_____
    2. Telephone_____ How many?_____ Locations:_____
    3. Lifeline phone_____
  D. Bathroom
    1. How many?_____
    2. Toilet: Height from floor to seat:_____ inches
    3. Location: Ground floor_____ Second floor_____
    4. Width of door:_____ inches
    5. Width of room:_____ feet_____ inches
    6. Bathtub: Yes_____ No_____
    7. Type of bathtub (on legs; new style):_____
    8. Shower: Yes_____ No_____
    9. Is wall of such construction that a railing could be attached if necessary? Yes_____ No_____
    10. Are faucets easily usable? Yes_____ No_____
  E. Kitchen
    1. Size of kitchen (approx. no. of feet):_____
    2. Please diagram the placement of the major appliances, e.g., refrigerator, stove, sink.
    3. Cabinet height from floor to lowest shelf:_____
    4. Stove: Electric_____ Gas_____
  F. Family rooms (give name, size, and location)
    1._____
    2._____
    3._____
  G. Bedroom
    1. Location: Ground floor_____ Second floor_____
    2. Width of door:_____ inches
    3. Size of rooms:_____ feet (e.g., 9 x 12 feet)
    4. Height of bed:_____

principles of therapeutic exercise. When working with the client who has an emotional disability, the family may be asked to watch for any acute signs of distress or changes in behavior or feelings. The multidisciplinary team may develop mechanisms for monitoring the client's status on a daily basis after discharge. Examples include exercise programs with simple illustrations, flow charts for documenting exercises to be done, medication schedules, and diet instruction materials. Homemakers and home health aides are trained to work with the client. When possible, the client is taught to convey to others those techniques and principles that are most effective in assisting him.

Community resources may be introduced by the occupational therapist so that further contacts are made directly by the family. The family may also be encour-

OCCUPATIONAL THERAPY HOME ASSESSMENT FORM—CONT'D

H. Carpeting: Wall-to-wall______ Area rugs________

I. Is there special equipment already in the home (e.g., grab bar, commode, wheelchair)? Please list and include location by floor:

J. Type of car used for transportation of client:
2-door________ 4-door________ Van ________

II. *Describe the client's probable function after discharge in the following areas:*

A. Self-care activities:

B. Homemaking activities:

C. Child care activities:

D. Recreational activities:

E. ADL communication:

F. Employment:

G. Describe any transportation or driving requirements or difficulties:

H. Is patient safe in an emergency?

1. Accessible phones:
2. Emergency numbers:
3. Fire escape:
4. Lifeline phone indicated:

I. Who will be available to assist the client in the home (individuals and community resources)?

III. *Describe the following:*

A. Family roles:

B. Client's self-image:

C. Family strengths:

D. Family weaknesses:

IV. *Goals to be achieved before discharge*

A. For the client:

B. For the team:

V. *Specific recommendations* (will be typed separately and sent to client and family):

EQUIPMENT	REASON	METHOD OF ACQUIRING

Signature of therapist:

aged to monitor the client's exercise and medication schedules and to identify architectural barriers that may prevent the client from achieving maximum independence. National health agencies such as the Arthritis Foundation and the Multiple Sclerosis Society offer valuable services to clients and families.

Prevocational training and adjustment to job placement. The occupational therapist determines whether a client with a physical or emotional handicap is to return directly to employment, or whether a day care center, sheltered workshop, or special education center is indicated. A prevocational assessment by the therapist may

RESTAURANT ACCESSIBILITY EVALUATION FORM

Name of restaurant: ______
Location: ______
Type of restaurant: ______
Price ranges: ______

I. *Parking*
   A. Wheelchair parking? Yes ____ No ____
   B. If so, distance from parking to building: ______
   C. If not:
      1. If handicapped parking plates are used, is alternate parking available? Yes ____ No ____ Where? ______
      2. What possibilities are there for parking without difficulty? ______

II. *Access to building entrance*
   A. Ramps? Yes ____ No ____
      1. Location: ______
      2. Length: ______
      3. Angle: ______
      4. Type (i.e., is it intended for wheelchairs or loading): ______
   B. Curbs? Yes ____ No ____
      1. Location: ______
      2. No. that must be traversed: ______
      3. Height: ______
   C. Pavement
      1. Type (e.g., concrete, brick, cobblestone, gravel): ______
      2. Slope: ______
      3. Comments: ______

III. *Entrance*
   A. Steps? Yes ____ No ____
      1. How many: ______
      2. How high: ______
   B. Threshold? Yes ____ No ____ Height: ______
   C. Door
      1. Type (e.g., swing in or out, revolving): ______
      2. Width: ______
      3. Weight: ______
      4. No. of doors in entrance way: ______
      5. Height of doorknob: ______

IV. *Inside*
   A. Aisle width: ______
   B. Floor covering: ______
   C. Table height: ______
   D. Table type
      1. Counter: ______
      2. Booth: ______
      3. Separate tables: ______
   E. Seat type
      1. Stools: ______
      2. Fixed chairs: ______
      3. Movable chairs: ______

include career choice inventory, evaluation of cognitive and perceptual-motor skills, communication abilities, hand function, and ADL skills. The client's potential for driving a vehicle and all psychosocial issues are also explored.

The occupational therapist may confer with an employer about a client's need to discuss any adjustment difficulties that the client or co-workers may experience. It is important to ensure that a particular task or responsibility suits the physical abilities and psychological framework of the client without being overwhelming.

RESTAURANT ACCESSIBILITY EVALUATION FORM—CONT'D

F. Stairs? Yes_____ No_____ How many: __________
G. Elevators? Yes_____ No_____
   1. Location: __________
   2. Elevator control height: __________
H. If salad bar
   1. Height: __________
   2. Aisle width: __________
   3. All areas reached from chair? Yes_____ No_____
I. Bar
   1. Tables: __________
   2. Bar and stools: __________
   3. Stairs: __________
   4. Waitress service: __________
   5. Self-service: __________
J. Cash register
   1. Height: __________
   2. Width of aisle: __________
K. Telephones? Yes_____ No_____
   1. Height: __________
   2. Location: __________
L. Bathrooms? Yes_____ No_____
   1. Location: __________
   2. Door width: __________
   3. Threshold: __________
   4. Stall door width: __________
   5. Toilet height: __________
   6. Sink height: __________
   7. Are there specially designed stalls for wheelchairs? Yes_____ No_____
   8. If so, describe: __________

V. *Attitudes*
   A. Were employees helpful when obstacles were confronted? Yes_____ No_____
   B. Was interest shown in wheelchair accessibility? __________
   C. Comments: __________

VI. *Can special arrangements be made?* Yes_____ No_____
   If so, describe: __________

For example, the handicapped client in a wheelchair or with limited mobility skills should not have a position in which satisfactory job performance is inhibited by architectural barriers.

Homemaking skills. In the occupational therapy clinic, homemaking training sessions are directed at setting goals with the client to meet the anticipated mobility level the client will need after discharge. The client is taught to maintain a balance between activity and rest and to manage work and energy efficiently. Adaptive equipment in the kitchen for meal preparation and the performance of all housekeeping skills is introduced. The occupational therapist may use the home evaluation forms (pp. 164-165 and 172-173) during home visits.

Planning for discharge to an extended care facility

When the multidisciplinary team has made the final decisions about the discharge plans and goals with the client, placement in an extended care facility may be necessary. The occupational therapist can contribute to a smooth transition for the client and family and assure the other team members that a specific placement setting will meet the individual needs of the client. Making site visits prior to the discharge date is recommended. It is important for the occupational therapist to understand the frame of reference of a facility as well as to determine what level of care and services are offered. Meeting the staff of the facility provides an opportunity to discuss the client's needs, abilities and limitations. The occupational therapist may determine whether the extended care facility has marked architectural barriers that are different from those of the institution where the client is presently staying. If such problems are present, the occupational therapist may review the client's functional status prior to discharge to determine whether new techniques or additional services or devices are necessary. It is important that the multidisciplinary team discuss the facility with the family and client to identify all concerns.

DOCUMENTATION OF DISCHARGE SUMMARIES AND REFERRAL WRITING

Documentation of discharge summaries serve several purposes: evaluation of continuity of care, protection of accreditation, maintenance of supervisory control, participation in research, and compliance with laws affecting the defense of a claim. A sample discharge summary appears on pp. 177-178. Abbreviated language, except a standard or universally accepted abbreviation, is often a source of confusion for other health care providers and should be avoided. Discharge summaries may include at least the following items:

1. Client identification information
2. Client's course of treatment and response to it
3. Indications and contraindications to therapy and functional abilities
4. Functional status at discharge (including the client's *physical* status as it relates to abilities and limitations)
5. Goals initially established and those achieved at discharge (including reasons for not meeting some goals)
6. Discharge plans (placement, level of care required, home exercise program, assistance of family and support systems, equipment required, etc.)

The use of discharge summaries is also recommended because additional referral information can be included. Essentially, discharge summaries differ from referral forms in that discharge summaries contain more information about the client's *course of treatment and response to it,* whereas referral forms are a synopsis of the discharge summary. When a referral is being made, the discharge summary and additional information—for example, specific instructions on the care and use of assistive devices—should be included.

OCCUPATIONAL THERAPY DISCHARGE SUMMARY

Client name:____________________ I.D. number:________________
Admission date:____________________ Discharge date:________________

Mrs. Tobey is a 73-year-old woman with osteoarthritis who was admitted to General Hospital for medical stabilization after a fall. She suffered a T-12 paraplegia, resulting in lack of sensation, tone, and muscle control below the lesion. She has had some difficulty in adjusting to her recent disability. In addition, her accident has left her with urinary incontinence. After discharge, Mrs. Tobey will be going to live in Oval Park, a handicapped housing unit in Manhasset (near her home town). As before her accident, she will be living alone.

RANGE OF MOTION AND MUSCLE STATUS: On admission, Mrs. Tobey's strength was good to good plus in her upper extremities. Both upper extremities have increased to "normal" strength as a result of a strengthening program. Her range of motion is within normal limits. Her endurance has increased greatly. Her grasp measures 45 to 50 lb on a dynamometer on both hands. She claims some mild pain on gripping, probably due to the arthritis, but there are no deviations in her musculoskeletal makeup at this time.

SENSATION: Sensation is within normal limits on the upper extremities. There are some deficits noted on the lower extremities, and further information on this matter is more detailed in the physical therapy discharge note.

PERCEPTUAL/COGNITIVE FIELDS: Perceptual fields and cognitive skills are intact. As noted there is some difficulty in Mrs. Tobey's psychological adjustment to her disability, and this is elaborated on later in this summary.

ACTIVITIES OF DAILY LIVING/FUNCTIONAL STATUS/SELF-CARE SKILLS:

Self-care: Mrs. Tobey is now independent in washing, dressing, and grooming at bedside. She can transfer to the tub with a transfer tub seat and one person to assist, stabilizing only. Transfers from the wheelchair to the toilet are independent with a head-on procedure and with the use of a guardrail on the right side of the toilet only. Dressing and undressing techniques were assessed, and several options have been suggested. Training in this area was no problem. Incontinence has been a large problem for Mrs. Tobey since her admission. A visiting nurse will see her for follow-up bowel and bladder training after discharge.

Homemaking: The client was given a lapboard pattern, which a relative will use to make a wooden lapboard for her. This item will enable the transfer of food from the stove to the table with safety and independence by the client. Kitchen activities that might be difficult after discharge were assessed with the client, and many problem-solving sessions were held. She was resistant to practicing a simulated homemaking situation in the OT clinic but was very cooperative when a home visit was made with this therapist. The purpose of this visit was to evaluate the home for any barriers that may arise during activities of daily living, and to introduce compensatory mechanisms.

Continued.

OCCUPATIONAL THERAPY DISCHARGE SUMMARY—CONT'D

Community mobility: Mrs. Tobey now transfers independently from wheelchair to car with the use of a sliding board but cannot care for her wheelchair after that. The client is mobile to wheelchair-accessible places due to training sessions on ramps, walkways, hallways, etc. The client does not drive.

COURSE AND RESPONSE TO TREATMENT/PSYCHOSOCIAL ATTITUDES: A concern of the occupational therapy goals was to support and facilitate realistic concerns for this client, who was not accepting her disability well and who spoke of "miracles" to allow her to walk again. Through repeated sessions in which the client was encouraged to vent her feelings of frustration and concern with the future, many gains were made in working toward appropriate decision-making and problem-solving skills. She has the intellectual ability and the physical strength to cope with problems she may encounter in her new living situation. Medical issues such as bladder control will be an obstacle for her, and she will need some outside support. She has been helped greatly by the few family members she has, and this assistance has been very beneficial for her in facing the future.

CONTRAINDICATIONS: There are no noted contraindications to therapy in relation to the medications Mrs. Tobey is receiving.

DISCHARGE PLANS: Oval Park Handicapped Housing Units were evaluated by the occupational therapist for accessibility. I believe the client will be able to function in her home well. She will require assistance for cleaning, laundry, and shopping. Her clergyman will coordinate friends, relatives, and neighbors to assist her with some activities. The social worker here may make a referral to the local Home Care Corporation for further support needs. A referral has been made to the Visiting Nurse Association for assistance with suppositories. Team meetings have been held biweekly to discuss these plans, and occupational and physical therapists have collaborated to develop a home exercise program for Mrs. Tobey. She may need counseling services later, and those family and friends who have come to the hospital for teaching sessions have been advised to monitor this possible need. Mrs. Tobey will be seen one month after discharge to review status and assess any new problems or needs.

EQUIPMENT RECOMMENDED: Tub seat (transfer type), guardrail for toilet (right side only), lapboard pattern, and sliding board. Payment will be made through Medicaid for these items, and an order was placed for delivery and installation of equipment just prior to discharge.

OCCUPATIONAL THERAPY GOALS: All occupational therapy goals were met during Mrs. Tobey's stay at the hospital. They included the following:

1. Increase of bilateral upper extremity strength
2. Increase of endurance and tolerance level to physical activity
3. Assessment and training in areas of self-care and activities of daily living
4. Evaluation of community mobility potential and proper placement
5. Provision of psychological support

The client was discharged to her home on ______________________

Therapist: ______________________
Date: ______________________

After the client has been discharged from a program, the therapist rarely has the opportunity to evaluate his own discharge planning efforts. For professional growth, and to advance the skills and knowledge of each therapist, the use of internal audits and written feedback mechanisms by client and family or referral agency is suggested. The client, family, or extended care facility, through the use of these mechanisms, will help the therapist evaluate his work and may highlight new considerations (e.g., community resources or architectural barriers).

SUMMARY

In summary, the occupational therapist brings to the multidisciplinary team the perspective of viewing clients as total human beings who will return to a community or proper placement setting and meet the demands of the environment as independently as possible. A presentation has been made to highlight the components of the discharge planning process and to suggest some occupational therapy tools to aid in this process.

The occupational therapist utilizes several tools when planning discharge for a client, including structured simulated environments, assistive devices, community field trips, and the introduction of community health agencies for postdischarge support.

There are four major considerations in the discharge planning process: client participation, the expertise of the multidisciplinary team, the use of community resources, and the influence of the family or significant others.

I encourage colleagues in the profession to publish expanded material on discharge planning criteria for specific disabilities, so that standard operating procedures may be established.

ACKNOWLEDGMENT

I wish to thank Valerie Williams, B.S., O.T.R., for her assistance in organizing the original structure of this paper, and Frances Portnoy, Ph.D., of Boston State College, for her wisdom, encouragement, and time in aiding the preparation of the manuscript.

READINGS

Fidler, G. S., and Fidler, J. W.: Occupational therapy: a communication process in psychiatry, New York, 1963, Macmillan Publishing Co.

Mosley, A. C.: Activities therapy, New York, 1973, Raven Press.

Spackman, C. S., and Willard, H. S., editors: Occupational therapy, ed. 4, Philadelphia, 1971, J. B. Lippincott Co.

CHAPTER 14

Discharge planning: a speech-language pathologist's perspective

LILLIAN WEINER GRAY

This chapter introduces the speech-language pathologist and explains what services professionals with training offer to the patient and health care team. An important message of this chapter is that early intervention by a speech-language pathologist in cases of communication problems has advantages for all concerned and should be encouraged. It is also suggested that the speech-language pathologist be called when the multidisciplinary team, in working with a patient who has communication problems, must consider decisions regarding diagnosis, management, or discharge planning.

The steps of the discharge planning process are discussed in relation to the role the speech-language pathologist can contribute, both as a primary care giver and as a consultant. (Information about the distribution and availability of speech-language pathology services is discussed.)

Speech-language pathologists are the health care professionals with special training and expertise in human communication, its normal development, and its disorders. Professional speech-language pathologists can be identified by their holding a Certificate of Clinical Competence from the American Speech, Language, and Hearing Association. Certified speech-language pathologists are the members of the health care team who are qualified to offer assistance to persons with speech and language disorders.

The role of the speech-language pathologist varies greatly with the needs of the particular work setting. Usually, however, the following services are provided:

1. Diagnosis and treatment of individuals who have disorders of articulation (speech sounds), voice, rhythm, and symbolization (language)
2. Counseling of patients and their families regarding the communication disorder

3. Initiation of referrals to other disciplines when appropriate
4. Instruction of health care workers and educators in the principles of speech and language development and disorders
5. Participation in multidisciplinary team evaluations, program planning, and discharge planning

Since discharge planning presupposes an admission, this discussion will begin by focusing on the patient with a communication problem who is in the acute hospital. The most commonly seen communication disorders in the acute hospital include aphasia, dysarthria, apraxia (usually as a result of stroke or brain trauma), neurogenic muscular disorders (Parkinson's disease and multiple sclerosis), voice disorders (nodules, polyps, paralysis), and cancer-related disorders (laryngectomy, hemiglossectomy, brain cancer).

The training of speech-language pathologists permits them to provide important services to the acutely ill, hospitalized patient with a communication disorder. The profession as a whole strongly urges early intervention. In hospitals with an active speech-language pathology department, early intervention usually takes place.

The physician generally requests an evaluation of the patient's problem. Treatment and counseling are then initiated. In hospitals with a speech-language pathology department the nursing staff encourages the physician to obtain a speech-language evaluation when a referral is not forthcoming. However, there are a large number of hospitals across the country that do not have speech-language pathologists affiliated with them in either staff or consultant positions. In these hospitals the health care workers, families, and patients are neither afforded the benefit of early diagnosis, treatment, and counselling nor given advice regarding long-term management and discharge planning.

CONTRIBUTIONS OF THE SPEECH-LANGUAGE PATHOLOGIST AS A PRIMARY CARE GIVER

The speech-language pathologist makes several contributions to the discharge planning team. First, the patient's level of communication is assessed and transmitted to the team. This information assists the team in determining the appropriateness of a home-alone disposition. Second, the patient's potential for improvement in communicative functioning through further treatment is determined, and recommendations are made to the team. The speech-language pathologist offers guidelines for the team in determining the degree of intensity required of services and the specific area of expertise the provider should possess. The speech-language pathologist usually has knowledge of colleagues in the community and can offer specific direction to the team.

Recommendations of the speech-language pathologist are combined with those of the other health care professionals on the discharge planning team. The final discharge plan is shaped by factors such as the patient's physical mobility and health status, transportation options, the patient's place of residence, his financial situation, and the wishes of the patient and family.

CONTRIBUTIONS OF THE SPEECH-LANGUAGE PATHOLOGIST AS A CONSULTANT

The input of the speech-language pathologist in planning the discharge of the communicatively handicapped patient can be valuable even though there has been no primary care given during the acute hospitalization. It is therefore recommended that discharge planning teams include consideration of the patient's communicative skills in the discharge assessment. Consideration should be given to how well the patient speaks, writes, understands, and reads. (A sample format for this information is shown below.)

When the discharge planning team identifies a patient who has communication difficulties, the skills of the speech-language pathologist can be used as a resource in planning for the patient's discharge. The consulting speech-language pathologist will assist the team by reviewing the patient's hospital record, screening the patient briefly, and making recommendations on whether the patient should have a speech and language evaluation and what type it should be. Frequently the specific area of expertise of the speech-language pathologist will be specified. The participation of a speech-language pathologist in the discharge planning assures the patient and family that expert advice was sought.

Some acute care hospitals have neither speech-language pathologists nor a department affiliated with the institution. In such cases the discharge planning team may choose to locate a speech-language professional in the community, who could act as a resource consultant to the discharge team. An appropriate place to locate

INVENTORY OF COMMUNICATIVE SKILLS

Language spoken by patient: ____________________

MODALITY	NO DIFFICULTY	IMPAIRED ABILITY*	NO FUNCTIONAL ABILITY*	PATIENT AWARE-NESS OF PROBLEM	FAMILY AWARE-NESS OF PROBLEM
Speaking					
Writing					
Understanding					
Reading					

*Indicate whether condition existed premorbidly.

such a resource person is through the state speech and hearing association, the professional group for speech-language pathologists and audiologists.*

The resource professional can act as a telephone consultant for the discharge team. This consultation offers the discharge team guidance in seeking services for the patient.

PROCESS OF DISCHARGE PLANNING

It is recommended that the speech-language pathologist be a part of the discharge planning team for all patients with communcation problems. Where the speech-language pathologist has been a primary care provider to the patient, the role is clearly defined. In cases where no speech-language pathologist has been involved with the patient, the discharge planning consultant should call on the resource or consultant speech-language pathologist for advice in planning a communication rehabilitation program for the patient. Where no resource or consultant speech-language pathologist is available at the time of discharge planning, the discharge planning team may plan for the patient to have a speech-language evaluation after discharge, at a facility that offers services. Plans for a communication rehabilitation program must then be postponed until the results of the evaluation are known.

The discharge planning process can be viewed as following natural, progressive steps. In this process, information is collected, problems are identified, plans are formulated and implemented, and outcomes are evaluated.

Assessment and diagnosis

The speech-language pathologist assesses the patient's communication disorder, makes a diagnosis, and relates it to the patient's discharge. The patient's communication disorder is rated by severity relative to functional level of communicative independence. The potential for improvement in communicative function is determined. Short-term and long-term goals for an intervention program are defined. Specifications for an optimum treatment program are offered in terms of type of service, intensity of service delivery, duration of services, and appropriateness of setting in which services will be received.

---

*This group can be located by contacting the parent body, the American Speech, Language, and Hearing Association, 10801 Rockville Pike, Rockville, Md. 20852. The Association publishes the *Guide to Clinical Services in Speech Pathology and Audiology,* which lists all known facilities in the United States that provide services for speech, language, and hearing problems. Programs are listed as accredited or nonaccredited by the American Board of Examiners in Speech Pathology and Audiology. Listings are by state and city. Descriptions of the size of the program, the types of disorders treated, the referral sources that are acceptable, and the name, address, and telephone number of the program director are included. The guide also lists certified speech-language pathologists and audiologists who are in private practice. The American Speech, Language, and Hearing Association also publishes a directory, which lists its membership alphabetically and by city and state.

Planning

Within an acute hospital environment the patient seen by the speech-language pathologist is always known to physicians and nurses. The patient may also be involved with physical and occupational therapists, nutritionists, and social workers. It is generally with this group of professionals and the patient and family that the speech-language pathologist shares responsibility for formulating a discharge plan.

The team is usually faced with the following options in planning for discharge:

1. Home alone without continued services
2. Home alone with continued services
   a. Home health services
   b. Outpatient services
3. Home with family
4. Rehabilitation hospital (Veterans Administration hospital for those qualified)
5. Skilled nursing facility
6. Long-term care at either a chronic disease hospital or a nursing home

The speech-language pathologist carefully considers the options for intervention relative to the patient's health, mobility, family situation, transportation, and third-party coverage. (A chart of the speech-language services available at various discharge sites is shown below.)

AVAILABLE SPEECH-LANGUAGE PATHOLOGY SERVICES

SERVICE SITE	MEDICAL REFERRAL REQUIRED	USUAL INTENSITY OF TREATMENT	TRANSPORTATION REQUIRED	GROUP TREATMENT	INDIVIDUAL TREATMENT	OTHER REHABILITATION SERVICES AVAILABLE
Acute hospital outpatient	Yes	1 or 2 times weekly	Yes	Yes	Yes	Yes
Rehabilitation hospital outpatient	Yes	Daily	Yes	Yes	Yes	Yes
Veteran's Administration outpatient clinic	Yes	Varies	Provided	Yes	Yes	Yes
University training clinic	No	1 or 2 times weekly	Yes	Yes	Yes	Yes
Home health agency	Yes	1 or 2 times weekly	No	No	Yes	Yes
Private practitioner	No	Varies	No	No	Yes	No
Long-term care facility	Yes	1 or 2 times weekly	No	?	Yes	Yes

Options that are considered for delivery of speech-language services after discharge from an acute hospital or rehabilitation hospital usually include the site where the services will be delivered, the type of service required, the intensity of service required, and the availability of services.

Site where services will be delivered. The speech-language pathologist may deliver services at the following sites:

1. Outpatient ambulatory clinic in acute hospital
2. Outpatient department of a rehabilitation hospital
3. Outpatient department of a free-standing, independent speech and hearing center
4. Outpatient department of a university speech and hearing student training center
5. The client's home

Type of service to be delivered: The speech-language pathologist offers the following types of services to the client:

1. Group treatment only
2. Individual treatment only
3. Combination of group and individual treatment
4. Treatment in conjunction with other health care professionals

Intensity of service required. The intensity of speech and language services varies among the various discharge sites. In choosing a particular placement for post-discharge care, the discharge planning team should be aware that in most cases the frequency with which communication rehabilitation will be available to the patient is automatically included in that choice. Increasing the intensity of treatment usually accelerates the improvement that patients make in treatment. Generally, daily treatment sessions are recommended for patients with newly acquired disorders that significantly interfere with communication.

Availability of services. The availability of speech-language pathology services varies greatly across the country. Generally, metropolitan areas are better served by speech-language pathologists than rural areas. The availability of speech-language services also varies among facilities according to the level of care permitted by a facility's license. The following discussion explains the variations in service available in terms of levels of care.

Within rehabilitation hospitals. Rehabilitation hospitals generally have a department of full-time speech and language pathologists. Patients are usually evaluated promptly after admission to the hospital and are seen daily in treatment. The speech-language pathologist functions as a member of the patient's rehabilitation team and is active in case finding, goal setting, counseling, and discharge planning. Since speech and language functions are overlayed on primary life support systems (mastication, respiration, etc.), recovery usually takes a longer time than the patient's stay in the rehabilitation hospital. For example, the speech and language treatment for stroke patients commonly lasts six months to one year after onset.

Since the typical length of stay in a rehabilitation hospital is eight to ten weeks, the speech-language pathologist will have to plan for continued speech and language treatments after discharge. The advantage to the patient of the two- to three-month stay in a rehabilitation hospital is the intensity and coordination of services available. Both intensity and coordination accelerate the recovery process. It is anticipated that by the time discharge is made from the rehabilitation hospital, the need for such intensive services will be diminished.

Within skilled nursing facilities. The role of the speech-language pathologist in the skilled nursing facility (SNF) is varied and not easily characterized. All SNFs are required to have speech-language pathologists. However, the method with which they offer these services varies, and therefore each specific SNF must be investigated. There are some SNFs where daily speech and language services are available to patients. These facilities generally are large enough to support rehabilitation staff or to subcontract services from an agency such as the Easter Seal Society.

More commonly, SNFs contract with individual speech-language pathologists to become consultants to their patients. Consultant contracts are often on a fee-for-service basis. The relationship of the speech-language pathologist is to the patient directly and not to the facility. The consultant, under this type of contract, would not be reimbursed for time and energy spent in team planning, staff education, discharge planning, or case screening. Since there is no regulated frequency of delivery of services by consultants in SNFs, great variety exists. Frequently, consultants to SNFs have their major employment within another organization and provide consulting services to SNFs on an irregular basis. The time available to treat patients may then be restricted, and services may be delivered only late in the day (not the optimum time for patient benefit). One final consideration when choosing consultant services in a nursing home is the availability of backup services during the consultant's illness or vacation.

Members of the discharge planning team should become knowledgeable about the type of speech and language services available at the various SNFs that are used in discharge planning and should coordinate efforts to see that patients with significant communication disorders are placed in facilities that can deliver the needed intensity of care.

Within a nursing home and at home. Some patients may be discharged home or to a facility that does not offer speech and language services. In either of these cases, arrangements can often be made to have the patient treated as an outpatient in a hospital speech and language department, independent speech and hearing center, or university speech and hearing clinic. If there are physical limitations and the patient is homebound, services may be obtained by a speech-language pathologist in private practice or through a home health agency. Since the availability of speech-language professionals varies greatly among facilities, the disposition of a communicatively handicapped patient is a heavy responsibility. A speech-language pathologist should be consulted about the service intensity that would be most appropriate for any particular patient.

There are many issues to consider when one is contemplating the feasibility of outpatient services. The patient must be mobile enough to transfer from the wheelchair to a car or taxi without physical assistance. In some cases the patient must be able to descend stairs independently or with minimum physical assistance. In some communities wheelchair vans are available from municipalities or civic agencies at a minimum cost per ride. These vans do not require that the patient move from the wheelchair when being transported. When transportation must be by private chair cars or ambulance, thought should be given to alternative home care services so that excessive costs can be avoided. A certain level of functional communicative skills appears necessary for the safety of patients who will be home alone awaiting taxis or chair cars to transport them to a center for outpatient treatment. Frequently these transportation systems experience delays or other scheduling changes. The patient alone at home needs to have the skills to telephone for information or assistance when these incidents occur. A nurse or physician should be consulted regarding the general physical health of the patient and the patient's ability to tolerate the physical and perhaps emotional stress of leaving the residence for services.

A great advantage in selecting an outpatient service site is the support that can be gained by the patient and family by being with other patients and families in a similar situation. Another advantage of some service sites is that the services of the various disciplines that will be involved with the patient can be obtained from one agency, thus facilitating team planning and cooperation. The services of many disciplines are usually available at outpatient hospitals or outpatient rehabilitation centers and sometimes through multidisciplinary home health agencies. Such services are less frequently available at free-standing speech and hearing clinics or in university speech and hearing training programs. Speech-language pathologists in private practice usually function without formal association with other disciplines.

The financial situation of the patient and family must also be considered in treatment-site selection. Financial coverage for services is often limited to certain types of providers, agencies, or sites of service delivery. Speech-language pathologists and discharge planning consultants should be familiar with the type of insurance the patient has and what limitations on coverage exist. Many patients will have no coverage or will have only partial coverage for speech-language pathology services. In these cases a clear understanding of what the patient and family can afford and are willing to spend is necessary. The speech-language pathologist should be knowledgeable about the charge structures of the various service delivery options in the community and should educate other team members. There are times when it is not possible for a patient to receive services within the *medical* care delivery system. Without a physician's referral, speech-language services cannot be reimbursed via many third-party programs. In such cases, however, when speech-language services are still desired, they may be obtained outside of the medical model. Services are available, without physician referral, from the speech-language pathologist who is a private practitioner or from a university training program. There are some patients whose insurance program does not provide adequate coverage for speech-language services and who cannot afford to pay for services privately. For these patients a clinic with a sliding fee scale or a university training program may offer less expensive alternatives.

Implementation. The speech-language pathologist has the responsibility as a primary care giver to make a direct referral to colleagues when continued speech and language treatment is appropriate. This responsibility does not vary with different discharge dispositions.

For patients who will be going to skilled nursing facilities or to chronic disease or rehabilitation hospitals with established speech-language pathology services, the role of the referring speech-language pathologist is twofold: (1) to promptly forward diagnostic reports and summaries of treatment to colleagues in the receiving facility and (2) to forward a description of the communication problem, together with suggestions for optimizing communication between the patient and the nursing staff. (This latter function can usually be accomplished by writing the information on the interagency transfer referral form.)

Patients whose disposition is to a long-term care nursing home present greater difficulties for the speech-language pathologist who is making referrals. It must first be determined whether the facility has a speech-language consultant. This information can be superficially determined by consulting listings in various nursing home guides. However, more accurate, up-to-the-moment information can be acquired by telephone contact with the nursing home itself. This telephone contact also presents an opportunity to determine who the consultant is, with what frequency patients can be seen, and what services are offered (e.g., group treatment, individual treatment, consultations with nursing staff).

The picture becomes more complicated if consultant services are not already established at the facility. The speech-language pathologist now has two options: (1) assist the facility in locating a colleague in the community who would be willing to provide services to the patient at the nursing home or (2) arrange for the patient to be treated in a hospital outpatient speech-language department. The former option often meets with some problems in the area of financial reimbursement to the consultant. The latter requires that transportation for the patient be arranged. When outpatient services will be used, the speech-language pathologist or other team members can investigate transportation alternatives, including family assistance, Medicaid taxi services, and civic or private shuttle services for the disabled and elderly.

For patients who are discharged home with home health agency support, it is not uncommon to find a speech-language pathologist on the agency's staff. Referral to the agency is accomplished in the same manner as to a facility with a depart-

DISCHARGE PLANNING AND FOLLOW-UP QUESTIONNAIRE

On __________, we referred the following patient, ____________________,
to your agency for services in the following departments: ______________

____

____

So that we may better understand the continuity of services we have planned for our patient, we would appreciate your completing and returning this form.

1. Did you have contact with the patient as planned? Yes _____ No _____
2. Was the patient's condition as expected from the referral information? Yes _____ No _____
3. Was this patient appropriate to your agency? Yes _____ No _____
4. Did you experience any difficulties with this referral? (Explain a yes answer, please.) Yes _____ No _____
5. Are you now continuing to provide services for this patient? Yes _____ No _____

Please estimate the length of time that services will be required by the patient:

____

ment. When the home health agency does not offer speech and language services, it is the responsibility of the speech-language pathologist to search among colleagues for someone willing to treat the patient at home. The success of this search depends on the proximity of the patient's residence to a speech-language pathologist as well as the financial mechanism available to reimburse for services. Today's unfortunate reality is that when services are reimbursed at a rate not appropriate to the community standard (as sometimes occurs with Medicaid), professionals are reluctant to offer home services.

Patients who are discharged home and are not homebound may, of course, be referred to a selection of outpatient facilities (including the acute hospital's own speech-language pathology department). In this latter situation, third-party coverage and transportation mechanisms are usually the focus of problems that arise.

Evaluation. It is often difficult to provide follow-up of patients who have been referred to other agencies for continuation of treatment. Some agencies send a summary note to the referral source when they have discharged a patient, but many do not. It may be useful to discharge planning teams, in evaluating the discharge plans they have made with the patient, to contact the patient, the patient's family, or the recipient agency. This contact might include a questionnaire similar to the one shown above, which is used for agency contact.

SUMMARY

The ability to communicate differentiates human beings from other animals. When this ability is lost or impaired, we are removed from the circle of man. The degree to which we are removed or isolated is proportional to the severity of the communcation disorder. Persons who are isolated by an inability to communicate often lose their will to live.

The speech-language pathologist is the most appropriate member of the health care team to determine the extent to which a patient can benefit from the treatment of a communication disorder. Early intervention by the speech-language pathologist in cases of communication problems offers advantages for the patient, the family, and the health care team and should be encouraged. The speech-language pathologist has important contributions to make to the discharge plan for patients with communication problems. These professionals should be sought out for advice if they are not readily available.

ADDITIONAL READINGS

Breaking the silence barrier: in-service training program, Washington, D.C., 1977, American Speech and Hearing Association.

Love, R., and Webb, W.: With equality for all? Convention presentation, Washington, D.C., 1978, American Speech and Hearing Association.

Schow, R. L., and others: Communication disorders of the aged: a guide to health professionals, Baltimore, 1978, University Park Press.

Stranberg, T. E.: A national study of United States hospital speech pathology services, report no. 1, ASHA **19**:69-76, 1977; report no. 2, ASHA **19**:160-163, 1977.

CHAPTER 15

Discharge planning: a community health nurse's perspective

KATHLEEN THOMPSON BURKE

The community health nurse (CHN) is frequently requested to implement discharge plans that originate when a client is hospitalized. The quality of the discharge plans may substantially facilitate or impede the initiation of community health nursing care. The CHN is in an excellent position to evaluate their effectiveness. Discharge plans made by the primary care providers are evaluated on the basis of their ability to communicate pertinent, current client information and to foster collaboration in the provision of continuous health care. The CHN uses discharge plans in providing nursing care to individual clients and their families in the home environment and in coordinating the delivery of home health services, including home health aide care, physical therapy, occupational therapy, speech therapy, social work services, and nutritional counseling.

According to the American Nurses' Association, community health nursing is

> a synthesis of nursing practice and public health practice applied to promoting and preserving the health of populations. . . . Health promotion, health maintenance, health education, coordination and continuity of care are utilized in a holistic approach to the family, group and community. The nurse's actions acknowledge the need for comprehensive health planning, recognize the influences of social and ecological issues, give attention to populations at risk and utilize the dynamic forces which influence change.[1]

Continuity of care, the ideal that health care providers strive to attain, is directly influenced by two major factors: *communication* and *collaboration*. It is recognized that these concepts are intimately connected; collaboration occurs only where positive communication exists. However, they are considered so essential to the success of discharge plans that the elements of each will be examined separately. One should be continuously aware of their interdependence.

Communication is the link joining the three parties involved in the discharge planning process. These three parties are the client and the client's family, the primary providers who make discharge plans, and the CHN. Communication with the client and the client's family in preparation for home care strongly influences the implementation of discharge plans. Effective communication, both verbal and written, between the primary providers and the CHN is essential to the success of discharge planning.

The CHN does not function in isolation but, rather, relies on collaboration with the multidisciplinary team of health care providers. Collaboration entails working together cooperatively to achieve a common goal. It should begin at the time of the client's admission to the facility and extend throughout the time care is provided by the CHN.

COMMUNICATION: THE LINK JOINING CLIENT, FACILITY, AND COMMUNITY HEALTH NURSE

From the perspective of the CHN, communication is the essence of discharge planning. It becomes the vehicle that carries discharge plans, both verbal and written, to the CHN for implementation. Although professional communication has a profound impact on the successful implementation of discharge plans, communication with the client is also essential. Unless the client and family are included in the planning process and are well prepared for home care, the implementation of discharge plans will be impeded. The CHN must rely on the primary providers to ensure that communication with the client has occurred.

Communication with the client in preparation for home care

The change from hospital to home environment can be greatly facilitated by communication with clients and families prior to discharge, preparing them for home care. The transition process from hospital to home care is often stressful for clients and families. They are asked to leave the protective atmosphere of the hospital, where they may have developed trust in the staff. At home they must adapt to a new set of health care providers. They will be expected to more fully utilize their own resources, since professional care will be available only on a part-time basis.

The establishment of the home care plan relies heavily on the client's and family's understanding of home care and their agreement to participate in the formation of the discharge plan. The patient has the ultimate right to accept or reject the plan. Without the cooperation of the client and family the efforts to initiate home care are futile. The CHN often depends on the family members to provide support and participate in the plan between visits; therefore it is essential for the family to be included in the planning stage. The client's confidence in the CHN will be enhanced if the client is certain that essential information has been communicated by the primary nurse. Little and Carnevali[4] have reiterated that some of the tension of moving may well be reduced if the client is aware that facts about patterns of activity and living, need, and preferences are being communicated to receptive listeners in the new agency. A predischarge meeting attended by the client, family, primary care providers in the facility, and CHN may ease the transition.

While explaining home care to the client and family, the primary provider responsible for coordinating discharge planning should consider cost. It is unfortunate that all necessary home health care is not covered by third-party insurers under the present system. The client should be made aware of the situation and should be advised that the CHN will discuss it more fully.

Verbal communication with community agencies

In addition to the written referral, the verbal sharing of information, via the telephone, is an effective method of communicating discharge plans to the CHN. A telephone call by the primary care provider ensures that information is relayed as quickly as possible. If one waits for a written referral to be received at the community agency, there is often an unnecessary delay in the initiation of home care services. In addition to the timesaving advantage of verbal communication, Little and Carnevali[4] believe that "verbal interchanges have the faculty of strengthening the bonds of communication and sense of responsibility between nurses in the agencies." In other words, verbal interchanges produce a more active participation in continuity of care.

From the perspective of the CHN it is essential that all pertinent information be conveyed during the telephone conversation because initial home visits are often made on the basis of information received at that time. Naturally the most complete information is communicated by the professional most familiar with the client's needs. Therefore the telephone contact should be made by the client's primary health care provider—usually, but not exclusively, the primary nurse. The primary nurse who assumes responsibility for providing holistic care for clients, including discharge planning, is well prepared to communicate complex, pertinent information and is able to knowledgeably answer questions regarding the client's care. Ideally, communication between nurses occurs at this time; that is, the primary nurse communicates discharge plans directly to a CHN.

In institutions where primary nursing is not practiced, the team leader, head nurse, or other designated person usually makes referrals. This person is responsible for gathering information about the client from available sources and relaying it to the CHN. Realistically, care providers with the most complete client information are not always available. An unanticipated discharge may occur when the person most familiar with the client is off duty. For this reason it is essential that facility nurses communicate with each other and clearly document a clent's nursing care. Whenever possible, an effort should be made to avoid referrals made by a person who barely knows the client and is unfamiliar with the client's care.

The person making the referral should provide the CHN with the names of all professionals who formulated the discharge plans, because clarification of information received in the telephone referral may be necessary. The CHN is often requested to implement physician's orders and must know the name of the primary physician and how to contact the person. Physicians are often difficult to locate. When more than one physician has been caring for a client, the names and specialities of each should be included. This policy will eliminate the possibility of contacting a client's physician only to be told that the question does not fall within that physician's jurisdiction.

In general, all referrals initially communicated by telephone should contain certain essential ingredients. *Identifying data* include the address and telephone number where the client will be residing after discharge. An incorrect address is often given because the person making the referral is unaware that the client is staying with relatives or friends after discharge. *Description of the client's health* is a succinct picture of the client, including physical, social, and psychological status at the time of discharge. The reason(s) for the referral should be clear, and the procedures to be done by the CHN should be fully explained. *Medications* are those the client is instructed to take at home and any medications with specific effects that are being given in the hospital (e.g., chemotherapy).

Written communication with community agencies

The written referral elaborates on information communicated in the verbal interchange. Multidisciplinary input into the written referral is essential to the communication of the total client picture. Each professional discipline that provided care to the hospitalized client has useful information to include in the written referral. Under the present health care system, care provided by a certified home health agency must be under the supervision of the client's physician; therefore a section of the written referral must contain the physician's instructions for home care and bear his or her signature. This constitutes legal physician orders and is necessary for third-party reimbursement.

A written referral containing pertinent information that can be utilized as a basis for the home care plan aids the delivery of cost-efficient care. Home health agencies, along with other health care providers, are seeking ways to curtail the rising cost of health services. If the CHN can avail herself of data collected during hospitalization, duplication of effort will be avoided and consequently costly time will be saved.

The CHN needs a written referral that is concise, complete, and organized. Answers are sought to the following questions: For what reason(s) has the referral been made? What are the multidisciplinary diagnoses indicating the need for home care? What are the nursing plans, nursing goals, and plans of other disciplines at the time of discharge? What information about the client is pertinent to the delivery of coordinated health care in the home environment?

The style of writing contributes to how well the information in the referral is understood. The paragraph format may contain pertinent information but is often lengthy and cumbersome. The problem-oriented method, on the other hand, employs a clear and organized style. Since many home health agencies utlize problem-oriented recording, information can be easily transferred to the agency record when a problem-oriented referral is received. Problem-oriented referrals communicate nursing information most clearly when nursing diagnoses are used as the problem statements. The CHN must document the need for care before receiving third-party reimbursement. The use of nursing diagnoses clearly indicates those entities the CHN is requested to treat. When nurses state the medical diagnosis as the problem requiring nursing intervention, confusion as to what exactly the nurse is doing often ensues. For example, a nurse does not give treatment on the basis of the medical diagnosis of fractured hip but on the basis of nursing diagnosis of alteration in mobility (caused by a fractured hip), and nursing intervention is planned to treat the altered mobility. Communication is facilitated when a common taxonomy is used, limiting the possibility of misinterpretation. For this reason some agencies are employing the National List of Nursing Diagnoses.[3]

In addition to medical and nursing diagnoses, professional diagnoses made by other disciplines should be included in the written referral. These diagnoses should be clearly stated, along with subjective and objective data. Concise statements of both the problem and the anticipated goals of therapy aid the formulation and implementation of the total home care plan.

Faulty communication leads to faulty discharge planning

If discharge planning is well done, the cycle of continuity of care continues unimpeded. Unfortunately, the CHN does encounter instances of faulty discharge planning, often caused by faulty communication patterns. Necessary communication has not taken place, resulting in the client's being discharged without the means to cope with postdischarge nursing needs.

Clients who have returned home with nursing needs that cannot be met by the family and who have not been referred for community health nursing care fall into two categories. In the first category are the clients and families who attempt to cope as well as they can; however, energies often become exhausted, which leads to rehospitalization. Hopefully, this will alert the hospital nurse to initiate discharge planning that will meet the client's needs at the time of the next discharge.

The second category contains clients and families who in a sense do their own discharge planning by contacting the CHN for assistance. When directly contacted by the family or client, the CHN must backtrack to obtain essential information. Often it is a prime concern to locate the physician so that pertinent medical information can be obtained. The facility that discharged the client must be contacted for nursing and multidisciplinary information. The task of locating information is often time consuming and frustrating, particularly if the client has been home for a length of time. Precious time elapses while necessary information is gathered and before a complete home care program is operative. The clients and families who contact the home health agency themselves eventually have their needs addressed, although there may be a delay. However, it is disconcerting to imagine the plight of clients who are not referred for home care and who may be unaware of whom to contact for assistance. Faulty communication in discharge planning can be remedied only by primary care providers who have access to discharge planning consultation and are able to anticipate the postdischarge needs of clients and to initiate appropriate referrals.

COLLABORATION BETWEEN COMMUNITY HEALTH NURSES AND PRIMARY PROVIDERS MAKING DISCHARGE PLANS

Productive communication cannot take place unless there is continuous collaboration between the CHN and the primary providers who formulate discharge plans. Collaboration is defined as "a cooperative endeavor in which the goals of patient care are clearly defined, known and accepted in the best interest of the patient."[5] It is not limited to the care of an individual client but rather is an ongoing effort of working together to achieve continuity of care for every client.

Continuity of care is facilitated when the CHN is recognized as a member of the multidisciplinary team of health care providers. This recognition occurs when the CHN is included in such events as predischarge planning conferences and team conferences. The liaison responsibility of a CHN in a facility fosters collaboration with primary providers and with the hospital discharge planning department.

Collaboration tools for discharge planning

The CHN is a generalist with a broad base of nursing knowledge and skills in addition to a special understanding of community resources. The CHN cannot be expected to have in-depth expertise in all hospital specialty areas; for example, the CHN may not be completely familiar with untoward effects of the most recent chemotherapeutic drugs. Therefore, if discharge planning is being done with a client whose care requires an exceptional amount of specialized knowledge and skill, the primary provider coordinating the discharge plans should initiate a predischarge planning conference. A multidisciplinary conference provides an opportunity for the entire team (including the client, if possible) to meet together for the purpose of sharing information and finalizing plans. If a complex dressing or other procedure is part of the client's care, the CHN may be able to observe the procedure at this time. Viewing the procedure provides a baseline for comparison so that normal can be differentiated from abnormal when the client is at home. The opportunity for the client to meet the CHN prior to discharge may also serve to allay the client's anxiety.

Case 1. A predischarge team conference was held for a variety of reasons when John P., a 29-year-old lawyer with Crohn's disease, was scheduled for discharge. He had undergone surgery three weeks previously, which resulted in an ileostomy. Almost immediately after the operation he developed excoriated skin around the stoma. John's skin was extremely sensitive and reacted to many skin preparations. After much frustrating trial and error, Susan H., John's primary nurse, and the hospital's enterostomy nurse therapist found a treatment that was effectively healing the skin irritation, although the procedure was fairly complex. Susan had started teaching John the entire ileostomy care and, with John's permission, included his mother in the teaching plan. John lived with his mother, a widow. John described his mother as "well meaning but sometimes overprotective" and felt it would be helpful if she knew the ileostomy care. John was very methodical in his approach to the ileostomy care and requested that all his supplies be set in an exact order. He became frustrated if he could not get the appliance to adhere exactly as he desired. When he became frustrated, he refused to continue the care. When this happened, if his mother was present, she would want to "take over" and complete the care. Susan had to frequently remind her that John had to be able to care for himself, and that her role was to assist when he needed a "third hand." Susan's long-range goal was for John to be independent in the ileostomy care.

When John was told by his surgeon that he was to be discharged in two days because he was progressing well, he became upset and demanded that the discharge be delayed. He turned to Susan and said: "How can you let them send me home? I'm not ready yet. You know I need a nurse near when I take care of this thing. What if I have a question? What if something goes wrong? I'll be right back in the hospital." Susan reassured John that he was ready to leave. He could manage the ileostomy care with minimum assistance from his mother, and the skin irritation was almost healed. She explained that, with his permission, a referral would be made and a CHN would visit at home. John's anxiety was not reduced. He declared: "I don't want a strange nurse to visit who doesn't know me or my problem. That's no help at all. Those nurses just know how to take care of babies—one visited my sister after she had a baby. I just can't go home yet. Maybe next week."

Susan conferred with the discharge planning consultant, and a predischarge conference was arranged for the following day. Susan spoke with the CHN prior to the conference, explaining John's anxieties. The CHN was introduced to John in his hospital room. The CHN explained that she had visited clients with ileostomies in the past and was familiar with their care. She explained that CHNs visit clients with all types of nursing needs, not just mothers and babies. Although the appliance did not need to be changed, at Susan's request John explained the steps involved when he performed the ileostomy care. The conference that followed was attended by John, his mother, Susan, the surgeon, the social worker, the nutritionist, the discharge planning consultant, and the CHN. John told them he still was apprehensive about going home the following day. Each member of the team emphasized the progress he had made, assuring him that he was ready to leave. They would be available via the telephone if problems arose. The CHN would telephone him at home the following afternoon and visit the subsequent morning. He would be given supplies to take home and the name of a local pharmacy that carried the appliance he was using. He was given written instructions that described the ileostomy care, and the CHN also received a copy. He already had received thorough diet instruction. After the conference Susan spoke to the CHN, describing approaches that had been successful with John and his mother. The CHN stopped by John's room before leaving to say that she looked forward to speaking with him the next day. He said that although he was still anxious, he realized the discharge would take place and felt relieved that someone who seemed competent would check in on him. The discharge took place as scheduled. The CHN telephoned Susan after the second home visit. John had changed the appliance with the CHN present, and no unusual problems had been encountered. A tentative team conference, scheduled to be held in two weeks, would be canceled if John continued to do well at home.

Collaboration also includes the responsibility of the primary providers to anticipate the client's immediate postdischarge needs. The CHN is able to change dressings and perform other procedures only when the necessary supplies are present. These supplies include dressing supplies, irrigating solutions, parenteral medications, syringes, and so on. Neighborhood pharmacies do not store a large selection of these supplies, and it is often impossible to obtain them on short notice. A three-day supply, sent home, is usually sufficient until the CHN assists the client in locating sources to replenish supplies.

Periodic multidisciplinary team conferences, held for the purpose of reviewing the progress of certain clients, are valuable tools for collaboration between the CHN and the primary providers who formulate the discharge plans. In addition to sharing information, team conferences provide the CHN with the opportunity to receive support and advice from the multidisciplinary team. In the interest of cost containment, some agency administrators may be reluctant to allocate time for the nurse to attend team conferences, under the premise that this use of agency time is nonproductive. However, in the long run, time may actually be saved when the team members put their heads together to find solutions to problems that have been impeding the client's progress and necessitating more frequent and lengthy home visits. The CHN should be expected to attend conferences when a client's needs are complex and there is a possibility that problems can be alleviated. If conference time absolutely cannot be spared, perhaps the nurse could be available to the team via the telephone. It should be kept in mind that team conferences are held for the client's benefit, and although cost containment is important, the client's well-being is our primary concern.

Providing nursing care in the community to a client with multiple complex needs can be a lonely experience. The nurse is often the sole health professional visiting the client and is responsible for the nursing care provided. Although a degree of support may be received from the community agency, being able to share feelings and discuss problems with professionals who are familiar with the client often lessens the burden. The awesome responsibility of caring for a terminally ill client or counseling a family with serious parenting problems is alleviated if a team of professionals participate in the planning of care and provide support.

Liaison role of the community health nurse

Collaboration between the CHN and primary providers of the facility is enhanced by the presence of a CHN liaison facilitator. This CHN is usually present in the facility on a regular part-time basis, depending on the needs of the facility, and serves as a bridge between the facility and the community, bringing community health nursing expertise and drawing on resources. The liaison role in the facility is unusual. The CHN acting in a liaison capacity serves within the facility, functioning as a member of its discharge planning department while being employed by the community agency and serving as its representative. Success depends heavily on effective use of interpersonal skills.

A key to success is the establishment of a workable relationship between the discharge planning consultants and the CHN. Their roles should be complementary, leading to a unique opportunity for collaboration. They share the common goal of continuity of care for clients requiring discharge planning but approach it from different perspectives, the discharge planning consultant from the perspective of the facility and the CHN from the perspective of the community. The discharge planning consultant needs to be assured that the CHN will not aggressively "take over" the department or infringe on the consultant's role. On the other hand, the

CHN acting in the liaison role is not a substitute to be called on when the department is unusually active or understaffed. The liaison CHN should contribute an added dimension to the discharge planning process.

As an outsider the liaison CHN must diligently work at becoming known to the staff of the facility, particularly nurses, physicians, and social workers. After initial introductions to the staff are made by the discharge planning consultant, the CHN is required to maintain contact. One means of achieving this goal is to attend discharge planning rounds, which are usually conducted regularly on facility units. When any situation arises in which the client would benefit by having community health nursing expertise, the liaison CHN must initiate the offer of consultation. The more familiar the staff becomes with the CHN, the more frequent will be their requests for consultation. If the CHN is intimidated by physicians or facility staff, valuable opportunities for consultation may be lost.

The primary nurse has ultimate responsibility for discharge planning and for making the referral for community health nursing care. As a consultant the liaison CHN is available to advise whether home care is appropriate for a particular patient. Questions can be answered about the availability of community resources and home care services. The focus of the liaison role is collaboration with the primary providers.

The presence of the liaison CHN in the hospital serves as a reminder to clients and staff that home health care is available. Home care clients who are currently hospitalized may be visited by the CHN to assure them that the nurse in the community is concerned and that home care will be reinstituted when they return home.

The presence of the liaison CHN at multidisciplinary team conferences facilitates contact between the hospital and community. The CHN contributes current knowledge and expertise in the community health nursing area and represents the interests of the home health agency and the patients receiving home care.

The liaison CHN may also act as the coordinator of such special programs as the Coordinated Home Care Program of Blue Cross/Blue Shield. This program is designed to facilitate early discharge by providing intensive home care services to patients with complex needs. The liaison CHN assists in the identification of clients eligible for this special type of home care. The primary nurse maintains responsibility for the discharge planning, whereas the CHN is available as a consultant.

Achieving collaboration with health care providers in emergency room settings

From the perspective of the CHN, establishing lines of communication with the staff of the entire facility, including emergency room staff, is important. Unfortunately, the emergency room is notoriously the source of inadequate or inappropriate referrals. Communication received is often incomplete or inaccurate, which leaves the CHN unable to assess the seriousness of the client's condition. The problem CHNs have with emergency room referrals stems from inadequate discharge planning done during the emergency room encounter. Insufficient data collection leads to inaccurate assessments. The faulty discharge planning is not totally blamed on the emergency room staff but is fostered by the operation of the emergency system. The emergency room is necessarily crisis oriented. Client encounters must be as brief as possible, and priorities are constantly being reordered. The client either requires hospitalization or is quickly treated and sent home to make room for other arriving clients. Frequently, clients are referred with problems that either are outside the realm of nursing intervention or are more complex than was initially realized.

Collaboration by the CHN with health care providers of the emergency room is difficult because of the unique functioning of the emergency setting. When problems are complex and not easily solved, health care providers of the emergency room often do not invest the time required to collaborate with the CHN. The physician often does not take the risk of making decisions about the care of a client seen only once. Skilled social work is often not available to the emergency room for crisis intervention, and often the clients referred to the CHN have complex social problems.

Obviously it is the patient and family who suffer the most. Being shifted from one source of care to another without any apparent progression toward a solution must be extremely disheartening.

The following example of inadequate discharge planning from an emergency room will serve to illustrate the problem.

Case 2. A community health nursing agency received a referral from an emergency room nurse to visit Mrs. J., 81 years of age, who had been taken to the emergency room of a local hospital by her son the previous night. The referral reported that Mrs. J.'s blood pressure was recorded as 180/100 and requested the CHN to monitor the vital signs. An appointment had been made for the hypertensive clinic for the following week.

An agency nurse was given the referral and went to the address given. The nurse found Mrs. J. and her son in a small, dark apartment. Mrs. J. was wearing a tattered dress and was sitting up in a bed with soiled bedclothes. She was disoriented and emaciated. Her son told the nurse that he had been trying to care for his mother as best he could. He was unable to bathe or turn her or coax her to eat. He had taken her to the emergency room because he was no longer able to cope and felt that she would be better off in a nursing home. The nurse bathed Mrs. J., checked her vital signs, and told her son that an effort would be made to ease the situation.

Back at the agency, attempts by the nurse to contact the emergency room staff were fruitless. The nurse who had made the referral would not be working until the next day, and the physician had been a "moonlighter" who would not be back until the following week. After a number of telephone calls the discharge planning department was able to arrange hospital admission for a complete physical and psychosocial examination. The CHN had expended much energy in convincing the hospital personnel that it was unhealthful for Mrs. J. to remain in the home environment.

This example may seem dramatic but unfortunately is not unusual. Although avoiding these occurrences through proper discharge planning practices in the emergency room is not simple, some change is possible. Even the slightest improvement may prevent some unfortunate happenings.

Obviously the emergency room staff members cannot be expected to devote time to seeking thorough information from one client while another client is experiencing a life-threatening crisis. However, if more attention were given to discovering the underlying cause of a client's immediate problem, discharge planning would improve. Emergency room nurses who are more familiar with the role of the CHN will be better able to make appropriate referrals for community health nursing. This education could be done by the liaison CHN or by personnel from the discharge planning department. Information about the existence and function of community agencies that would facilitate referrals to more appropriate resources should also be given. Availability to the emergency room staff of both a discharge planning consultant[2] and someone skilled in crisis intervention may alleviate problems and ensure that appropriate assistance is provided. Simplest and perhaps most beneficial would be an attitude of willingness to communicate with the CHN.

SUMMARY

Discharge planning is extremely important to the practice of community health nursing. It is possible to provide quality nursing care in the community only when communication and collaboration with primary providers in facilities are maintained. It is the responsibility of the multidisciplinary team members, in the facility and in the community, to be continuously attentive to maintaining and improving productive relationships with each other. All members must guard against becoming so involved in their particular area that they lose sight of the broader responsibility for continuity of care.

REFERENCES

1. American Nurses' Association: Standards of community health nursing practice, Kansas City, Mo., 1973, the Association.
2. Brodnax, S.: Community health nurses as discharge planners. In Archer, S. A., and Fleshman, R. P., editors: Community health nursing: patterns and practice, ed. 2, North Scituate, Mass., 1979, Duxbury Press.
3. Gebbie, K.: Summary of the Second National Conference on the Classification of Nursing Diagnoses, St. Louis, 1976, Clearinghouse National Group for Classification of Nursing Diagnoses.
4. Little, D., and Carnevali, D.: Nursing care planning, Philadelphia, 1976, J. B. Lippincott Co.
5. O'Brien, M. J.: Communications and relationships in nursing, ed. 2, St. Louis, 1978, The C. V. Mosby Co.

ADDITIONAL READINGS

Beaudry, M. L.: Effective discharge planning matches patient need and community resources, Hosp. Prog. **56**:29-30, Dec., 1975.

Combs, P. A.: A study of effectiveness of nursing referrals, Pub. Health Rep. **91**:122-126, 1976.

Isler, C.: Helping hospital patients—out, RN **38**:43-46, Nov., 1975.

Jennings, C. P.: Discharge planning and the government, Superv. Nurse **8**:48-52, March, 1977.

LaMontagne, M. E., and McKeehan, K. M.: Profile of a continuing care program emphasizing discharge planning, J. Nurs. Adm. **5**:22-33, Oct. 1975.
Moreland, H. J., and Schmitt, V.: Making referrals is everybody's business, Am. J. Nurs. **74**:96-97, 1974.
Nikkila, M.: Securing early referrals for home care, Am. J. Nurs. **62**:58-60, 1962.
National League for Nursing: Patient discharge and referral system: whose responsibility, New York, 1974, the League.
Will, M. B.: Referral: a process not a form, Nursing (Horsham) **7**:44-45, Dec., 1977.

CHAPTER 16

Discharge planning: a nursing home administrator's perspective

LOUISE W. BRINE

My 44 years of experience as both a nursing home administrator and a nurse have taught me many things; however, the most important lesson I've learned is the value each patient places on personal *independence*. The greatest fault of both society in general, and health care providers in particular, toward the elderly in nursing homes has been a consistent failure to recognize this fact. That fault can, however, be eliminated if health care providers and society begin to recognize that nursing homes are an extension of hospital care. Permanent placement in a nursing home has the potential to drastically reduce personally perceived independence, remove a sense of purpose of life, and destroy the will to live. Facility placement does not always have to be viewed as a permanent setting for the patient. In those situations in which patients cannot return to their homes, the goal mutually set by the patient and facility personnel should be rehabilitation to the patient's maximum potential for functioning within the protective environment of the nursing home. Patients should be more involved in their own goal setting. This "positive control" over their own life can greatly enhance their sense of independence.

Physicians, nurses, social workers, and all allied health professionals have a serious obligation to consider the *patient's goals* when planning for discharge from one facility to another, or for discharge home. No one disagrees with this assertion, but surprisingly few health care providers actually act on it. My own philosophy is that every person has the right to hope for the achievement and maintenance of the highest possible level of health and function. Inherent in this philosophy is a reciprocal obligation on the part of all health care providers to ensure that patients receive the required help to attain their goals. Focus in nursing homes should be redirected from maintenance to some form of rehabilitation. This philosophy contradicts the prevailing assumption that the older a person is, the more inevitable permanent nursing home placement will be if that person becomes ill. Although the typically slow healing process in the elderly may necessitate transfer to an extended care facility or nursing home, this step should never be considered final and irreversible. Tragically, too many health care providers in all sectors of the system see no other alternative, thus confirming the elderly person's worst fears and guaranteeing an inevitable series of personal losses for him.

The primary responsibility of hospital and nursing home personnel in the discharge planning process is to carry out the goals of the patient. To adequately fulfill this responsibility, the coordinator of the discharge plan must effectively collaborate with the patient, significant other persons, and all members of the various disciplines involved in the patient's care. If one accepts the premise that nursing homes are ideally a temporary extension of health care rather than permanent residences, then planning for discharge from the hospital or nursing home becomes a dynamic process rather than a passive receiving event. This chapter will address the discharge planning process from two major transition points: (1) from an acute care facility (i.e., a hospital) to a nursing home and (2) from a nursing home to the community or back to the hopsital.

DISCHARGE PLANNING PROCESS

Discharge planning process from hospital to nursing home

Nursing home personnel rely heavily on the patient assessment provided by the transferring facility. Information on such items as the patient's diagnosis and the current medical regimen is usually provided routinely. These data, although important, tell us little about the individual as a person. Illness is an event in a person's life, and we need to know how it has affected the patient as an individual. To more fully appreciate this event, one must learn the patient's prior status with regard to living arrangements, support systems, interests, abilities, and work and activity patterns. It is also essential to consider what the patient most valued and appreciated before illness and to relate these facts to the patient's goals and desires for the future. Most patients who come to a nursing home are fearful. They are afraid of the things they have heard and read about nursing homes. Rarely do the news media, for example, tell about the accomplishments that nursing homes have achieved. Patients are afraid that they are not going to behave in the way that the staff members of the hospital or nursing home expect them to behave. They "clam up" and ask no questions because they do not want to be a burden. They try to behave in the way they think people want them to behave. On the other hand, some patients may exhibit antagonistic or belligerent behavior before discharge. It is important for hospital personnel to share an honest profile of the patient's behavior. The short period of hospitalization is not always long enough to determine all the causes of this behavior. It is important for health providers to think about how they might feel in a similar situation.

The staff in an acute care setting play a vital role in helping the patient to adjust to the nursing home transition. This requires that the staff view nursing homes as centers for extended rehabilitation where the objective is to help the patient to maximize his functional potential. It also requires that the staff develop a special sensitivity to the perceptions that elderly persons have of nursing homes. For example, many elderly persons harbor significant fears of such facilities because they seem to them to be places where one goes, helpless, dehumanized, and useless, to vegetate until death comes.

Nurses can easily reinforce the patient's strengths and abilities in the hospital setting by encouraging maximum participation in daily care and decision making. It is so easy to call a person by name, provide privacy, and display respect. Elderly patients lose their dignity quickly when their slowness interferes with a hospital's efficiency. Perhaps the greatest cause of the loss of dignity for the older person is incontinence, because it is associated with infancy, childishness, and degradation. The patient who is incontinent is often confused and considered senile because incontinence seems so degrading to the human being that the patient pulls down the curtain on reality. Although this condition is sometimes unpreventable during the acute phase of illness, there are few patients for whom bladder training cannot eventually work. Nurses who begin such regimens in the acute care setting must communicate their plans to receiving facilities so that the work begun can be continued, thus restoring dignity more quickly.

Hospital staff should involve patients in the decision-making process when a nursing home transfer is contemplated. Patients need "positive control" over their lives. Tools that enhance this positive control include brochures from the nursing home and invitations to personnel from the nursing home to meet the patient in the hospital. A good example of the utilization of positive control can be seen in the following case study of a patient in our nursing home.

Case 1. Mrs. C., an 80-year-old woman, had fractured her hip. The surgical repair of this hip required the first hospitalization in her life. I was invited to visit this patient in the hospital and talk with her regarding a possible admission to our nursing home. During our first meeting, Mrs. C. stated, "You are here to see if you want to take me, aren't you?" My response was, "No, I have come to see if you would like to come with me and if you feel we are going to do our utmost to help you go back to your own apartment." Immediately her attitude changed, and we began to plan her admission to our facility together.

After admission to our nursing home, Mrs. C. stated, "Now, don't get me out of bed, because I can't walk." I explained to her that she was not going to start to walk today, but that when she was ready, we would begin the rehabilitation program the hospital team had suggested. We convinced her that we would not force her to get up; however, she did consent to let us exercise her good leg and help her move in bed as much as possible. Good principles of rehabilitation nursing were utilized without aggressively forcing her into the planned regimen. A few days later she called me into her room and stated: "I don't understand. The other three ladies in this room are up and walking, and one of them had a fractured hip last year." I answered that she was right and that she, too, could walk, but not overnight. Mrs. C. then began to actively talk about her goal to walk again and eventually go home. From that point on, she was ready to help create and participate in her own rehabilitation program. Besides leg mobility, her plan included other activities of daily living, such as regaining expertise in the kitchen.

Patients coming to a nursing home exhibit many fears. They often do not know how to tell anyone what the fears are because they have kept their feelings bottled up inside of themselves for so long. Hospital and nursing home staff need to sit down with them and help them bring these feelings out into the open. The secret is loving them and having them know that you love them—letting them know that you care and will listen to them.

Finally, there is no more effective motivation in life than to feel useful and productive. By finding out how the patient met this need before illness, the staff can help the patient to determine how to continue to feel productive in the future. Once such a goal is identified, it is more likely that the patient will cooperate with, and participate in, a rehabilitation plan that includes nursing home placement. Clearly, the message here is to maintain hope; its power to potentiate our best efforts can be phenomenal, but its destruction will only hasten complications and death, and add misery as well. Experience has taught me to be cautious about labeling a patient's goal as unrealistic. Such judgments often prove to be wrong.

In conjunction with knowing patient concerns and fears regarding nursing home placement, staff members must also gain insight into patient behaviors and reactions that result from illness, enforced dependency, and threatened self-esteem. The underlying problem for the patient is the multiplicity of significant losses, both threatened and actual, with which the patient must continually cope. Except on an intellectual level, young, healthy, active, and independent health care professionals find it especially difficult to empathize with patients who have this problem. When staff members cannot determine the reason for angry, belligerent, hostile, or withdrawn behavior, it is important that they at least be honest in communicating that the behavior exists. The nursing home staff can then assess these behaviors more easily so that the etiology can be determined and effective intervention to reduce the patient's concerns can be planned.

Discharge planning process from the nursing home

The discharge planning process from the nursing home should begin during the patient's admission. The nursing home staff members should ask themselves the following questions: Where will this patient go when he is no longer in need of rehabilitation? When the maximum goal has been reached, can the patient return to the commmunity and live in his own apartment or with the family? How can we help the patient to function in the community? How can this elderly person become a vital factor in the home life he has left? Older people often feel that they have failed—failed because they grew old, because they became ill, or because they have lived longer than their loved ones and are now "alone." These feelings may be so intense that some patients may choose not to leave a nursing home to face the world and possibly fail again. They may need help to try new ways to socialize, such as joining a "golden age" group. Perhaps all their life they wanted to travel, and now they have no traveling companion. The question is, How do we start to motivate them to trust themselves and go after that resocialization? The answer often lies with the personnel in the nursing home. They have the opportunity to become well acquainted with these patients as individuals and to allow them to share the kind of wisdom that only age can bring.

Recreation groups in nursing homes give patients an excellent opportunity to begin the resocialization process. As an example of such an activity, a group in our nursing home created a "monkey doll." The doll was about 18 inches tall and was made from a huge sock that we stuffed with nylon stockings so that it was washable. Some of the patients cut up nylon stockings to make the stuffing, and someone else cut a stocking to make the arms and legs. Other patients sewed the various parts together, and still others stuffed the arms, legs, and body. Finally, the eyes, nose, and mouth were sewn onto the head. All the patients felt that they had had a part in making this particular item.

Case 2. For many patients, returning to the community is not an easy process. I remember one elderly gentleman who came to our nursing home, and on the bottom of the referral were the words "permanent nursing home care." Soon after his arrival the staff told me that he was in his room, crying. I went to his room, and he proceeded to tell me that he had been told that he had to give up all hope of ever returning to his home. This man was admitted to the nursing home for convalescence after having had pneumonia. When his physician was asked why this patient could never return to the community, the answer was that every year for the past five years, Mr. S. had developed pneumonia and had had to be hospitalized. The physician then proceeded to state that Mr. S. lived in one small room. Further investigation revealed that Mr. S. lived in a rooming house where the owners accepted him as one of the family. When he could not go out for a meal, they would invite him to dinner. It turned out that Mr. S.'s major problem was that he could not adequately manage the money he received monthly from Old Age Assistance. As a result, by the end of each month Mr. S.'s nutrition severely declined, and during the winter months he became highly susceptible to pneumonia. After Mr. S. was assured that our first goal was to return him to his room in the community, he enthusiastically worked with the nursing personnel on a plan to educate him regarding better nutritional habits and more efficient utilization of his money. This plan included accompanying Mr. S. to his local restaurant to share meals and review menus. Mr. S. was discharged from the nursing home and returned to his boarding house in the community, where he lived for two and a half years without further hospitalization. Every Sunday Mr. S. joined us at the nursing home for dinner. This contact provided an excellent opportunity for him to retain the friendships he had made, and it was important for other patients to see his progression back to the community as a future goal for themselves. It is difficult at times to convince physicians, nurses, and social workers that patients have the right to help define their own way of life.

Transition from the nursing home back to the hospital

There are times when a nursing home patient develops problems that require rehospitalization. The staff in the nursing home have a special responsibility here in carrying out the discharge planning process. In many ways the personnel in the nursing home have become a part of the patient's family. It is their responsibility to share the uniqueness of the patient with the hospital staff. A good example of what could happen during a rehospitalization is the experience of Mrs. W.

Case 3. Mrs. W., one of our patients who had had a stroke, did not have the ability to talk or swallow properly. Consequently, her food had to be of a specific consistency. It was important for the personnel in the hospital to understand that Mrs. W. had sharp intellectual capacities, even though she had lost her ability to express herself. At times Mrs. W. would become angry with herself and others.

She had been asked to leave a previous nursing home for throwing trays. When she came to our home, it was discovered that she could communicate through writing. Mrs. W. was precise in describing her wishes through her writing. For example, instead of just writing that she wanted tomato soup, she would qualify the term with the word "hot." She always ended her communication by writing, "I am an intelligent and well-educated individual." When Mrs. W. was transferred back to the hospital, she was accompanied by a detailed referral that reflected her needs and suggested approaches to meet her needs.

I visited Mrs. W. in the hospital one week later, and the nurses stated that she was not doing well at all. They elaborated on her refusal to participate in numerous activities, such as eating and walking. No one on the staff had attempted to carry out the suggested plans on the referral from the nursing home. As I approached Mrs. W.'s bed, she lay curled in a fetal position. When she saw me, she threw her arms around me and began to cry. I reassured her that she could return to the nursing home after she had demonstrated certain abilities to the hospital staff. Immediately we walked down the hall together, much to the amazement of the nursing staff. The point being emphasized here is that *discharge planning goals had not been set with Mrs. W. at the time of admission to the hospital.* She had lost all positive control over her own life, and her inability to vocalize her needs further intensified her limitations. She felt that her only recourse was withdrawal.

Communication through written referrals is vital, but communication does not take place if no one reads the assessment and suggested plan. So often, "approaches" to patient care are omitted from referrals. Staff at both hospitals and nursing homes need to know these approaches to help patients progress to the highest possible level of independence. We must allow patients to have more positive control over their lives. I have learned more from elderly people in my 44 years of nursing home experience than I have ever learned in any other mode of education. People are varied; we all think differently, hope differently, and desire differently. Many people do not truly believe that elderly persons have specific goals and desires, and often the goals and desires of others are imposed on them.

FACTORS THAT INFLUENCE PATIENT OUTCOMES IN NURSING HOMES

Many factors influencing patient outcomes in nursing homes affect the discharge planning process. In this chapter we will focus on four of the most important ones: (1) the knowledge deficit regarding the principles of gerontology in multidisciplinary education, (2) societal attitudes toward the elderly, (3) government rules and regulations affecting nursing homes, and (4) quality of care in nursing homes.

Knowledge deficit regarding principles of gerontology

Multiple disciplines within both hospitals and nursing homes need to understand more about the principles of geriatrics (the study of the ill elderly) and gerontology (the study of the normal process of aging). This could be accomplished by integrating the principles of gerontology into the curriculum of multidisciplinary education. Mobile in-service education programs could be presented in educational institutions, hospitals, and nursing homes, enabling staff and students to share their experiences and educate one another. Students in nursing, social service, and other disciplines should have the opportunity of field placement in nursing homes.

Societal attitudes toward the elderly

In the past, individuals believed it was their inherited responsibility to take care of elderly family members. Changes in society have made it difficult for individuals to care for elderly relatives. Some of these changes include the mobility of families, the employment of women, smaller homes, and inflation. If a nursing home placement is necessary, family members often feel guilty that they could not care for their relative. Nursing home personnel have a responsiblity to help families work through these guilt feelings.

Government rules and regulations

The government sets down rules and regulations controlling the environment—for example, in the areas of sanitation, food, and documentation of care. However, the nursing home has the responsibility to integrate the regulations in such a way that a homelike atmosphere is created for the patient. Since the government regulators do not live or work in the nursing home, it is difficult for them to understand the importance of this integration. The individuals who write the regulations usually have the best intentions of providing a safe environment for the patient; however, the regulations are often misinterpreted by individual inspectors who emphasize enforcement rather than a cooperative effort *with* nursing home personnel to achieve changes together. Furthermore, various regulations come from different departments in the state or federal government. It would be helpful if these departments communicated with one another on a regular basis. It would also be helpful if they utilized nursing home personnel as consultants to regulatory committees.

Quality of care

Nursing homes should determine their philosophy of care and then select personnel who believe in that philosophy. Nursing personnel who work in long-term care facilities need a strong commitment to quality patient care. Their patient population has far less turnover and, in some ways, may offer less stimulation than the acute hospital population. On the other hand, nursing home personnel have the opportunity to see patients achieve goals over long periods of time. Acute hospital personnel rarely have this opportunity and would benefit from feedback from nursing home personnel regarding the progress of their patients.

SUMMARY

In summation, discharge planning involves *communication* and *coordination*. Health care professionals should learn to work together as a team and with the patient to facilitate appropriate planning. Nursing home placement should be viewed as an extension of hospital care, enabling patients to experience rehabilitation to reach their highest functional potential. Patients should be actively involved in setting their own goals. The primary responsibility of hospital and nursing home personnel in the discharge planning process is to help the patient carry out these goals. Patient assessment and the sharing of approaches to plans of care are vital factors that may enhance the transition process of patients between hospitals, nursing homes, and the community. Many patients could return to the community if there were adequate support services available. The development of discharge planning programs in health care settings can do much to promote cooperative planning. Hospital and nursing home staff need to educate themselves further in the principles of gerontology.

ACKNOWLEDGMENTS

I would like to acknowledge two individuals who had a great influence on my career as a nursing home administrator: Rose Hallaren and John J. McNally.

Rose Hallaren was the administrator of Elm Hill Nursing Home, where I worked as a nurse's aide over 50 years ago. It was with her example and through her encouragement that I went to nursing school for the purpose of taking her place when she retired. I remained the administrator of Elm Hill Nursing Home for 44 years.

John J. McNally, R.N., M.D., came to America from Ireland at the age of 14 years. He was both a registered nurse and a practicing physician. His profound knowledge of people and the process of aging greatly influenced my professional career.

Appendixes

APPENDIX A

Annotated bibliography

ELIZABETH J. NEVEL

The purpose of this annotated bibliography is: to provide the reader with over 20 years of literature that explains rationales, processes, problems, populations, and needs inherent in the discharge planning process.

The selection of articles and books for the annotated bibliography was made from computer searches. The principal system utilized was the National Library of Medicine (NLM: 1969-1979). Literature in this retrieval system included articles from *Index Medicus, Social Sciences Citation Index,* and hospital and nursing literature. A Catline search (1966-1979) included books and serials from the NLM system. Other computer searches included *Excerpta Medica* (1975-1978), *Psychological Abstracts* (1967-1979), and the National Technical Information Service (NTIS: 1964-1979). The searches were done under the title heading Discharge Planning. Searches under other title headings, such as continuity of care, home care, aftercare, quality assurance, or utilization review, did not uncover enough material on the topic of discharge planning, or there was too much extraneous material.

The searches were augmented by the inclusion of titles from an annotated bibliography on discharge planning compiled by August La Rocco. The articles are dated from 1944 to 1968.

The annotations for the bibliography are arranged in three sections. The first section relates to the *rationales* for discharge planning. These articles contain information that focuses on the need for discharge planning, such as studies of patient outcomes and legal implications. Section two includes articles that present *profiles* of discharge planning programs. The third section of the bibliography includes articles that present *tools* or *skills* that can assist in the discharge planning process.

RATIONALES FOR DISCHARGE PLANNING

American Hospital Association: Reviewing the issues, Chicago 1977, the Association.

A brief review of four studies that indicate the need for discharge planning is presented. Thirteen references are reviewed as to the history and the present redirection and focus in discharge planning by hospitals. Four factors, (1) initiation of new staff members, (2) multidisciplinary planning, (3) intersetting experiences, and (4) inclusion of family members, are summarized for the development and maintenance of a discharge planning program.

Beaudry, M. L.: Effective discharge planning matches patient need and community resources, Hosp. Prog. **56**:29-30, Dec., 1975.

In a question-and-answer format the author cites the need for communication in obtaining accurate and comprehensive medical care and the need for leadership and creativity in obtaining and identifying postdischarge community services. The existence of government and third-party payers underscores the importance of discharge planning as a means of reducing health care costs. Nursing homes, home health agencies, hospital home care, and drop-in centers are presented as options for discharge planning.

Bristow, O., Stickney, C., and Thompson, S.: Discharge planning for continuity of care, New York, 1976, National League for Nursing, 143 p.

The authors present a series of discharge planning ideas and activities that have been developed by discharge planners. These planners are from throughout the United States and have experience in hospital, nursing home, home care, ambulatory, and long-term care settings.

Summaries of regulations that influence discharge planning, such as PSRO and utilization review regulations, are presented. Excerpts from programs such as *Selected Institute Papers: Spotlight on Patient Discharge Planning* enhance the sequential-step format for determining discharge planning needs and defining the functional roles of the discharge planner.

The appendix includes referral and follow-up forms, a discharge planning checklist, and a summary of responses to a questionnaire on discharge planning that was sent to hospitals and selected nursing homes in Virginia in 1974. An extensive bibliography is included.

Collier, J.: Hospital discharge planning: a hospital's responsibility to the patient and the community, J. Tenn. Med. Assoc. **66**:1037, 1973.

Because of societal cultural changes, organized health care should assume more family and community responsibilities for patient needs arising after discharge from acute care settings. A discharge planning team meets weekly to evaluate and determine goals for patients with potential postdischarge needs. The team consists of nursing supervisors, dietitians, social workers, and, when indicated, the physical therapist, respiratory therapist, or chaplain. The minutes of the meeting communicate the recommendations of the team to the primary physician.

David, J., Hanser, J., Madden, B., and Pratt, M.: Guidelines for discharge planning, Thorofare, N.J., 1973, Charles B. Slack, 59 p.

The authors, from Ranchos Los Amigos Hospital, have prepared a guidebook to assist nurses in discharge planning. Criteria for adults who could benefit from discharge planning are listed and enhanced with patient care examples. Aids presented that can assist the nurse in the discharge planning role include nursing care plans, referral forms, and a home layout form.

Department of Community Health Services, School of Public Health: Coordinated home care training manual, Ann Arbor, Mich., 1966, the School, 104 p.

The manual presents suggestions for planning and organizing a home care program, including guidelines for roles of both administrative and multidisciplinary participants, for services to be rendered, and for areas of program function that should be evaluated. Suggested readings and references augment the content provided.

Fell, P. E.: Home visits to evaluate planning, Am. J. Nurs. **79:**1452, 1979.

A one-month trial home visiting program was conducted by primary nurses from a coronary care unit. The results of a one-time home follow-up for 16 patients and the assessments and recommendations to improve discharge planning for patients are presented.

Hanser, J., Pross, E., Oechslie, F., and Reeder, L.: Continuity of nursing care from hospital to home: a study of a voluntary general hospital, pub. no. 11-1058, New York, 1966, National League for Nursing, 241 p.

A study in a Los Angeles general hospital describes outcomes as they are related to varied role methods used by a nurse for patient discharge planning. Statistics from the three-year study include the prereferral and referral time frames and the type of patient that benefited from aftercare. Underutilization of the community health nurse by hospitals is documented. The study relates to adult medical and surgical patients. A section of the study evaluated postdischarge care needs for a sample of emergency maternity patients.

Izsak, F., Engle, J., and Medalie, J.: Comprehensive rehabilitation of the patient with cancer: five-year experience of a home-care unit, J. Chronic Dis. **26:**363, 1973.

This article reports the first five-year experience (1965-1970) of a home care unit at Donolo Hospital in Yaffa, Israel.

A physician and social service home visit and the identified care needs of the patient provide the information for a multiprofessional team decision for the patient's use of the home care unit services.

Six short case presentations demonstrate the effectiveness of the unit. Statistics on patients and services are also presented. This comprehensive article illustrates that a focus on quality of life is also cost efficient.

Jennings, C.: Discharge planning and the government, Superv. Nurse **8:**48, March, 1977.

As the author explains components of federal legislation related to discharge planning, she espouses politcal awareness and responsibility by nurses to protect and to develop nursing practice. Legislation presented includes the 1972 Social Security Amendment, Public Law 93-641, and the National Health Service Corps. She encourages an awareness of legislation and regulations found in the *Federal Register,* Department of Health, Education, and Welfare.

Juntti, M. J.: Problem solving in arranging for comprehensive home care, Nurs. Forum **8:**103, 1966.

A case study of a chronically ill pediatric patient presents a vehicle for describing positive outcomes achieved by one nurse's thoughtful and comprehensive discharge planning.

Katz, S., Ford, A., Downs, T., and others: Effects of continued care: a study of chronic illness in the home, pub. no. 73-3010, Washington, D. C., 1972, Department of Health, Education and Welfare, 166 p.

This research study is an in-depth presentation of the effects of public health nursing on chronically ill, elderly people. Three hundred patients from a chronic disease rehabilitation hospital in Cleveland were followed for two years after hospital discharge. Interpretations as well as recommendations for directions in health care are presented.

Longabaugh, R.: The significance of a signicant other, QRB **2**:17, Oct., 1976.

A psychiatric facility used the Performance Evaluation Procedure for Auditing and Improving Patient Care (PEP) to determine the overall effectiveness of discharge planning. Discharge planning was reviewed for timeliness, comprehensiveness of the discharge plan, implementation of the plan, and success of the plan. An audit for discharge of psychiatric patients is presented. A study of the audit showed that patients who had a significant other person involved in discharge planning did better after discharge than those who did not.

McGuire, H.: Better continuity needed, Hospitals **50**:87, April 1, 1976.

The continuity and coordination of health services from a 1975 literature review revolve around trends and issues concerning use of personnel, effects of regulations, use of home care, and controversies over the use of the medical model. Nineteen references are cited.

Montefiore Hospital Association of Western Pennsylvania: Spotlight on patient discharge planning: developing guidelines for patient discharge planning, Pittsburgh, 1970, the Association, 193 p.

This book was compiled from two institutes presented in 1969 that focused on discharge planning as a first step toward ensuring continuity of patient care. The institute faculty consisted of social workers, physicians, nurses, and hospital administrators who held and shared deep convictions toward responsibility and multidisciplinary interaction for discharge planning for the benefit of the patient. Issues presented included (1) stimulation of community interest and response in postdischarge care, (2) guidelines for discharge planning from each discipline's point of view, (3) discharge needs of selected patient groups (geriatric, psychiatric, pediatric), and (4) implications for education of health professionals.

Murphy, F.: Blocked beds, Br. Med. J. **1**:1395, May 28, 1977.

A cross section of patients in a surgical ward after 28 days of hospitalization were assessed for nursing, social service and medical input. Thirteen percent of the acute beds were found to be blocked because of inability to transfer patients for further care. Twenty-eight percent of the patients had no plans for discharge. The author cites the need for teamwork so that each discipline will plan and implement follow-up care from the time of hospital admission, especially for the elderly person living alone.

National League for Nursing: Patient discharge and referral planning—whose responsibility? pub. no. 20-1515, New York, 1974, the League, 73 p.

Papers presented at the Patient Discharge and Referral Planning workshop in Birmingham, Alabama, in 1973 cite the views of assorted health professionals toward discharge planning. Community health nurses and a hospital nurse describe the use of and the need for communication and nursing services as two issues that influence the process of postdischarge care. A hospital administrator focuses on the hospital as a community health center that provides responsibility and leadership for postdischarge services and resources. Problems and issues of nursing home management and aftercare transfers to the facility are presented by a nursing home director. Other presentations discuss the relationship between discharge planning, PSROs, and payment mechanisms for hospital aftercare.

Pryer, M., and Distefano, M. K.: Short-term follow-up evaluation of a rehabilitation program for multiple-readmission psychiatric patients, J. Community Psychol. **1**:180, 1973.

An evaluation at Central Louisiana State Hospital revealed that symptomatology improved through a program that emphasized family and community involvement in treatment, discharge planning, and aftercare.

Rosenthal, J., and Miller, D.: Providers have failed to work for continuity, Hospitals **53**:79, May 16, 1979.

The authors indicate that their research demonstrates that interinstitutional transfer communication for patient care is inadequate. They present a description of a study on referral forms used to facilitate transfers from a hospital to a nursing home and vice versa.

Schuman, J. E., Ostfeld, A., and Willard, H.: Discharge planning in an acute hospital, Arch. Phys. Med. Rehabil. **57**:343, 1976.

This study documents discharge planning on one acute medical ward. The purpose was to evaluate the process and adequacy of its discharge planning. The authors concluded that discharge planning is often inadequate because of misunderstandings in diagnosis and treatment, failure to match the patient's aftercare environment with his needs, or lack of patient understanding toward his medical regimen. The authors suggest nursing service as the approach by which discharge planning can be improved. Twenty-four references are cited.

Simpson, J., Cox, A., Meade, T., and others: "Right" stay in hospital after surgery; randomised controlled trial, Br. Med. J. **1**:1514, June 11, 1977.

Surgical cholecystectomy and vagotomy patients were studied in groups of fixed-stay and right-stay discharge. The right-stay approach used in this study confirmed that there is a range of appropriate periods for postoperative stay in the hospital rather than a standard period applicable to all patients.

Stewart, J. E.: Home health care, St. Louis, 1979, The C. V. Mosby Co., 176 p.

Chapters 5 and 7 present the financial constraints on home care and the issues that ultimately influence home care delivery. Chapter 6, Continuity of Care, explains rationales for discharge planning and how planning can be done. The remainder of the book is an overview of the home health agencies in existence and the types of services they offer.

Tolkoff-Rubin, N., Fisher, S., O'Brien, J., and Rubin, R.: Coordinated home care: the Massachusetts General Hospital experience, Med. Care **16**:453, 1978.

Massachusetts General Hospital, an 1100-bed acute care Boston hospital, serves 30,000 inpatients and 300,000 outpatients annually. In 1968 the hospital entered into a coordinated home care (CHC) agreement with the Boston Visiting Nurse Association. The CHC, sanctioned by third-party payers, serves primarily the elderly, the chronically ill, and the terminally ill who require a variety of physical and emotional supports beyond the acute care setting. These CHC services prevent institutionalization, inappropriate use of hospital or long-term care facility beds, and inappropriate discharge to the community without adequate postdischarge care.

Cost analyses, length of stay, and service statistics are presented from the study of 800 patients who participated in the program. Three case reports demonstrate benefits of the program.

Vielhaber, C.: Accounting for social work activites in aftercare planning, Social Work Adm. **2**:2-5, Nov.-Dec., 1975.

A survey was conducted to account for the quantitative aspects of activities of social workers in discharge planning. The 1974 questionnaire included 22 northeastern Ohio social work departments in acute care hospitals. The author concludes that perhaps more questions were raised as a result of the survey than were answered. Survey questions included the number of days from admission to referral to social service, number of days from referral to hospital discharge, and number of days of medical readiness to actual patient discharge date. Other questions related to the hours used by social workers in service delivery.

Weinbach, R., and Dodge, D.: Educating for discharge planning, Hospitals **48**:72, 1974.

Regional workshops conducted by the South Carolina Hospital Association provided area hospitals with an opportunity to explore and develop discharge planning services. The exchange of ideas and information promoted useful professional relationships. Discharge planning, it was concluded, is not the exclusive function of any profession. It must be adapted to each hospital, its community liaison facilitators, and the services offered. Discharge planners, as leaders, can identify needs and coordinate services.

White, J.: Effective discharge planning can help reduce hospital costs, Utah Nurse **23**:24, Summer, 1972.

A summary of a study showed that referring patients for home nursing care is cost effective.

PROFILES OF DISCHARGE PLANNING PROGRAMS

American Hospital Association: Discharge planning for hospitals, Chicago, 1974, the Association, 26 p.

This booklet describes how to organize hospital discharge planning programs. The authors presume that there is a discharge coodinator and propose role responsibilities. Brief definitions of home health agencies, intermediate care facilites, skilled nursing facilities, rehabilitation services, and residential care are included. One third of the booklet presents the rationale and procedures for transfer agreements between general hospitals and chronic or long-term care facilities.

Chapman, A., and Harvey, A.: Making certain the patient understands: discharge planning nurse in the ED, J. Emerg. Nurs. **2**:33, March-April, 1976.

The emergency room is often the "access point" for health care. Beth Israel Hospital, New York City, utilizes a discharge planning nurse (DPN) to assess whether the patient understands and is able to follow through with the care initiated. The DPN, besides having had experience in emergency room nursing, is knowledgeable regarding community resources, communication and interviewing skills, and discharge planning goals. This approach promotes the integration of the patient into the health care system rather than the pursuit of emergency medical care. A case study and work sheets used by the DPN are included.

Edwards, R.: Professionals in "alliance" achieve more effective discharge planning, Hospitals **52**:71, June 1, 1978.

Professional alliance is described as nonterritorial complementary roles in which interacting professionals work to achieve responsible and responsive discharge planning services for patients. The "executive function" of discharge planners is to promote patient needs, resource systems, and the facilitation of services between individuals. The Methodist Hospital in Madison, Wisconsin, presents a general view of how social workers and patient care coordinators (nurses) interact to screen for, and follow through on, discharge planning needs.

Ferguson, K., Bowden, M. L., Lichinet, D., and others: Initiation of a quality assurance program for social work practice in a teaching hospital, Social Work in Health Care **2**:205, Winter, 1976-1977.

The University of Michigan Medical Center's social work department developed protocols for service delivery. The reasons for having protocols based on medical diagnosis or tasks rather than on psychosocial diagnosis are explained. The protocols offer a means for review, feedback, and evaluation of social service delivery. Protocols for adult discharge planning and adult nursing home placement are presented.

Habeeb, M. C., and McLaughlin, F. E.: Including the hospital staff nurse, Am. J. Nurs. **79**:1443, 1979.

Recognition by discharge planners of the staff nurse's knowledge of the patient adds to transfer information for a patient who is going to a nursing home. Other than checklist ADL information, the staff nurse's assessment of a patient's coping with illness, understanding of the reasons for transfer, and perception of the future, implied by convalescent care, adds broader dimensions to transfer information.

Hicks, A., and Ashby, D.: Teaching discharge planning, Nurs. Outlook **24**:306, 1976.

Senior students at Texas Woman's University have the educational experience of a three-week rotation as a home care coordinator. Activities such as interviewing, teaching, giving demonstrations, and contacting community agencies promote increased knowledge and leadership in discharge planning. The authors report that the students provided role modeling for discharge planning for hospital staff.

Hoff, B., Johnson, J., and Williams, T.: A psychiatric assessment unit for readmission screening in a VA hospital, Hosp. Community Psychiatry **28**:177, March, 1977.

The psychiatric assessment unit in the Salt Lake City Veterans Administration Hospital uses identification of patient stresses and support systems as factors for discharge planning. The use of community resources contributes to patient welfare and cost effectiveness.

Kieth, J.: Hospital social work audit focuses on discharge planning, Hospitals **51**:73, Dec. 1, 1977.

The social work department of a 600-plus bed hospital in South Carolina developed a discharge planning audit program. The article lists criteria for patients who are to be evaluated for long-term placement and describes an audit for comprehensive adult discharges. The audit provides a means to measure and evaluate professional social work services.

Kulys, R.: Discharge planning, Hospitals **44**:39, May 1, 1970.

A study by Holy Cross Hospital in Chicago was designed to identify possible discharge problems soon after patient admission. Discharge planning is facilitated through the use of a questionnaire. Patients who are 65 years of age and over are interviewed by personnel in the admitting department to obtain information on health, family resources, and living arrangements. The hospital's method of discharge planning and its multiple outreach services are also identified.

La Montagne, M., and McKeehan, K.: Profile of a continuing care program emphasizing discharge planning, J. Nurse Adm. **5**:22, 1975.

The authors provide a profile of the development and implementation of a discharge planning program at Boston Hospital for Women. The profile centers around 13 sequential guidelines utilized to create and implement a discharge planning program in an acute hospital setting. The article also includes a time framework for implementation, as well as recommendations and feedback from a questionnaire used to evaluate the initial stages of the program.

Moreland, H., and Schmitt, V.: Making referrals is everybody's business, Am. J. Nurs. **74**:96, 1974.

The philosophy at Mt. Sinai Hospital in Minneapolis is that discharge planning is best done by staff nurses who care directly for the patient. The hospital therefore has no discharge coordinator. The in-service education needed to implement this type of service is presented.

Previte, V.: Continuing care in a primary nursing setting: role of a clinical specialist, Int. Nurs. Rev. **26**:53, 1979.

The author shares her experience in developing and implementing a discharge planning program in a primary nursing care setting. She talks about her personal development during the transition from functional discharge planner to consultant for discharge planning to the nursing staff.

Sasano, E., Shepard, K., Bell, J., and others: The family in physical therapy, Phys. Ther. **57**:153, 1977.

Inpatients at the Stanford University Hospital and their families have the opportunity to live in homelike accommodations before hospital discharge. Through a program called Family Focus, the family members receive intensive training in the skills necessary for continuing the patient's care at home. The family or significant others are integral participants in achieving therapeutic goals for the patient. Through the predischarge trail period, the family members learn that either they can care for the individual at home or that other, more realistic alternatives must be chosen. The psychologist, as part of the team, assists in the approach to patient-family care through family dynamics assessment.

Schuman, J., and Willard, H.: Role of the acute hospital team in planning discharge of the chronically ill, Geriatrics **31**:63, Feb. 1976.

The continuing care unit at Yale–New Haven Hospital is a rehabilitation type of in-house unit. The multidisciplinary approach to patient care focuses on promoting optimum self-care and discharge to an environment that has adequate support.

Smith, J. A., Buckalew, J., and Rosales, S. M.: Coordinating a workable system, Am. J. Nurs. **79**:1439, 1979.

A nursing discharge planning program at the University of California at Los Angeles Medical Center, which was the responsibility of the utilization review department, is described as to implementation, duties, and outcomes.

Steffl, B., and Eide, I.: Discharge planning handbook, Thorofare, N.J., 1978, Charles B. Slack, 81 p.

The authors have prepared a handbook that contains generalized steps for the implementation of discharge planning. Also included are rationales for discharge planning, general managerial approaches, need for multidisciplinary teamwork, and possible roles for the team members. One chapter presents the seldom-written issues related to emergency room discharge planning.

Stephens, L.: Introducing a stoke service in a general hospital setting, Am. J. Occup. Ther. **29**:418, 1975.

Early identification of stroke patients who need rehabilitation is emphasized at the Morton Plant Hospital in Florida. The need for stroke service is initially identified through the admitting diagnosis. After one year of operation the original objectives of the program were met. They include (1) systematic identification of stroke patients, (2) support for families through social service and a spouse support group, (3) coordination of discharge planning, and (4) improved communication between various services. The utilization of the occupational therapy department increased over 50% in that year.

Thompson, H.: Assisting patients with post-hospitalization plans, Hospitals **47**:43, Jan. 16, 1973.

The discharge planning program at St. Francis Hospital in Evanston, Illinois, is based on three principles: the need for a multidisciplinary team approach; the conviction that continuity of care involves helping a patient with nonmedical as well as medical needs; and the philosophy that programs implemented by an institution are most likely to succeed when they are developed within the institution. The author includes information on how the program was planned and how patients are identified and receive postdischarge services. Services provided by the hospital to the community are enumerated.

Thoms, F. L., and Mott, R.: A new role for the RN: discharge coordinator, Hosp. Prog. **59**:38, 1978.

A social service author from St. Vincent Charity Hospital in Cleveland tells of the past professional service role provided to patients and their families. Patient placements in long-term care facilities were limited due to the lack of awareness of medical and nursing needs by social workers. The social service department added a registered nurse to facilitate the information and communication necessary for the transfer of patients to nursing homes. A follow-up study one year later indicated increased effectiveness in discharge planning.

SKILLS AND TOOLS FOR DISCHARGE PLANNING

*Abdella, F., Forest, H., and Chow, R.: PACE: an approach to improving the care of the elderly, Am. J. Nurs. **79**:1109, 1979.

Carefully planned efforts are needed to ensure quality care and containment of health costs associated with prolonged illness and long-term disabilities. The Patient Appraisal, Care Planning, and Evaluation (PACE) is a tool for systematic assessment of needed care and the effects of the care. It is patterned on a health care model rather than a medical model. The authors present an overview of the use and implications of the PACE tool. Parts of the tool will be utilized by the Patient Care Management System. This system will attempt to be used as a data source for administrative evaluation, measurement of quality of care, and appropriate patient transition in the health care system.

Barham, F.: Tentative program improves utilization, Hospitals **48**:83, Oct. 16, 1974.

The medical center at Princeton, New Jersey, devised a method to aid physicians in their responsibility for discharge planning. After three days of hospitalization, a stamp is placed on the patient's order sheet, requiring the physician to check the appropriate block for discharge services. The use of the stamp has accounted for an increase in (1) transfer to skilled nursing facilities for extended care, (2) use of the hospital-based home care program, (3) more referrals to social service, and (4) elimination of the crisis discharge situation.

Cucuzzo, R. A.: Method discharge planning, Superv. Nurse **7**:43, Jan., 1976.

The use of a tool known as METHOD (medication, economic, treatments, health education, outpatient referrals, and diet) provides an organized format for assessing, planning, and charting discharge planning data at Bronx Municipal Hospital Center. Comparisons of nursing notes in the narrative form and in the METHOD form present the difference in the quality of discharge planning chart documentation.

*Densen, P., and Jones, E.: The patient classification for long-term care developed by four research groups in the United States, Med. Care **14**(suppl.):126, May, 1976.

Four groups of investigators have collaborated to produce the Patient Classification for Long-Term Care. The classification identifies long-term care problems for adults and measures the effectiveness of efforts to deal with them. A summary of the patient classification descriptors is presented. The system is used to make objective, comprehensive, patient assessments both for a plan of care and for determining aftercare placement.

---

*Articles related to referral form research and construction.

*Department of Health, Education, and Welfare: Patient care management: theory to practice, pub. no. HSQB 78-010, U.S. Government Printing Office, 1978, 117 p.

A feasibility study on the PACE form provided this PACE II form. Besides the instrument, rationale for the patient appraisal data and guidance for translating the data into action through care planning and evaluation are included. PACE II includes the Minimal Data Set, which provides a means of collecting consistent data for all long-term care clients.

*Jones, E., Densen, P., and McNitt, B.: Assessing the quality of long-term care, no. 78-3192, Washington, D.C., 1978, Department of Health, Education, and Welfare.

An overview of the research at a chronic disease hospital and seven nursing homes demonstrates the use of the Patient Classification System for Long-Term Care. The system provides an assessment that aids in (1) planning patient placement and care, (2) measuring patient outcomes, and (3) developing standards for quality of patient care.

*Jones, E. W., McNitt, B., and McKnight, E.: Patient classification long-term care user's manual, pub. no. 74-3107, Washington, D.C., 1973, Department of Health, Education,. and Welfare.

This first attempt to systematize the information base of patients with chronic illness provides a tool for improving patient care. The classification is a patient assessment tool composed of descriptive terms that are patient oriented, multidimensional in content, objectively stated, precisely defined, and relative to the goals of long-term care. The authors state that classification provides the decision makers with uniformity of information but does not relinquish the professional judgment required for patient care and placement.

*Katz, S., and Akpom, A.: A measure of primary sociobiological functions, Int. J. Health Serv. **6**:493, 1976.

The index of independence in activities of daily living (index of ADL) has been used to provide predictive information about chronic conditions and to evaluate the benefits of long-term services. The index provides profiles of the behavioral levels of six sociobiological functions: bathing, dressing, toileting, transfer, continence, and feeding. The hierarchical nature of the functions enables comparisons to be made of rank and functional status among individuals or groups and provides the ability to detect change about the individual or group over time. As a screening measure and a survey measure, the index of ADL has offered information about health needs and outcomes that assist in management, planning, policymaking, research, and teaching.

Plovnick, M. S., Fry, R., and Rubin, I.: Managing health care delivery: a training program for primary care physicians, Cambridge, Mass., 1978, Ballinger Publishing Co.

Although this workbook-style presentation is oriented toward physician management, the focus on roles, interaction, and intercommunication addresses some of the basic problems inherent in coordination of care of which discharge planning is a component.

Rubin, I., Fry, R., Plovnick, M., and Stearns, N.: Improving the coordination of care: an educational program, Hosp. Health Serv. Adm. **22**:57, Spring, 1977.

---

*Articles related to referral form research and construction.

The importance of team management is presented for its effectiveness in the coordination of patient care. The authors present principles to examine, evaluate, and improve team management.

Rubin, I., Plovnick, M., and Fry, R.: Improving the coordination of care: a program for health team development, Cambridge, Mass., 1975, Ballinger Publishing Co., 279 p.

The book is designed as a group instruction guide for health workers and administrators who work as a team in delivering health care. Through seven three-hour periods of time, the group can explore and improve its effectiveness for setting goals and priorities, defining and negotiating roles, and analyzing decision-making processes. Optional guides include how to run a better meeting and how to develop leadership skills.

Ryder, C., Elkin, W., and Doten, D.: Patient assessment: an essential tool in placement and planning of care, Health Rep. **86:**923, 1971.

The history of patient evaluation that provides a system of assessment and classification for patient needs is reviewed by the authors and the need for such an evaluation is discussed. Patient assessment and classification are helpful tools that can be used in making decisions regarding patient placement within the health care system.

The authors use a model of patient flow to demonstrate situations in which the process of assessment aids in making decisions regarding the provision of health care services.

Three examples of patient assessment studies are presented. Issues related to validity and reliability of a patient assessment tool are discussed.

Stone, M.: Discharge planning guide, Am. J. Nurs. **79:**1446, 1979.

A questionnaire given to patients on admission assists nurses in the assessment, planning, and documentation necessary for discharge planning.

Vlack, J. E., and Connolly, M. G.: When a nursing home is the best choice, Am. J. Nurs. **79:**1450, 1979.

A dialogue between a patient in need of transfer to a nursing home and an acute care nurse illustrates the principles that can be used to prevent transfer trauma for the elderly patient.

SELECTED TITLES FROM AN ANNOTATED BIBLIOGRAPHY BY AUGUST LA ROCCO*

Altman, I.: Some factors affecting hospital length of stay, Hospitals **39:**68-73, July 16, 1965.

Anderson, E.: A continuity of care plan for long-term patients. In Lilienfeld, A., and Gifford, A., editors: Chronic diseases and public health, Baltimore, 1966, Johns Hopkins Press, pp. 186-191.

Bainum, R.: Preliminary steps to a hospital–nursing home patient transfer agreement, Hospitals **42:**78-80, June 16, 1968.

Bithell, J. F., and Devlin, H. B.: Prediction of discharge of hospital inpatients, Health Serv. Res. **3:**174-184, 1968.

*La Rocco, A.: Planning for hospital discharge: a bibliography with abstracts and research review, Boston, 1970, Harvard University Library of the Center for Community Health and Medical Care, 77 p. (Articles date from 1944 to 1968.)

Bliss, P.: Economics of rapid discharge from hospital, Br. Med. J. **1**:709, March 16, 1968.

Burstein, A. G., Soloff, A., Gillespie, H., and others: Prediction of hospital discharge of mental patients by psychomotor performance: partial replication of Brooks and Weaver, Percept. Mot. Skills **24**:127-134, Feb., 1967.

Clayton, G., and Entwistle, E. R.: Planned early discharge in Bradford, Midwives Chronicle **79**:342-343, Sept., 1966.

College of General Practitioners, Bradford Group: A survey of 100 early-discharge cases, Lancet **5**:536-540, March 5, 1966.

Commission on Chronic Illness: Chronic illness in the United States, vol. II: Care of the long-term patient, Cambridge, Mass., 1956, Harvard University Press, 606 p.

Craig, W. S.: Early morbidity among babies following discharge from a maternity hospital, Practitioner **197**:641-649, Nov., 1966.

Davis, M.: Discharge from hospital against medical advice: a study of reciprocity in the doctor-patient relationship, presented at the annual meeting of the American Sociological Association, Sept., 1965.

Donabedian, A., and Rosenfeld, L. S.: Follow-up study of chronically ill patients discharged from hospital, J. Chronic Dis. **17**:847-862, Sept., 1964.

Eberle, B.: A stochastic model for hospital admissions and discharges, Biometrics **23**:376, June, 1967.

Ewart, E.: The Canadian way, Bull. Natl. TB Assoc. **42**:171-172, Dec., 1956.

Fleming, W. L., Callahan, S. E., and Warren, S. L.: Service to discharged general hospital patients through local health departments, Am. J. Public Health **50**:779-784, June, 1960.

Fraenkel, M., and Erhardt, C. L.: Morbidity and the municipal hospitals of the city of New York, New York, 1955, Russell Sage Foundation, 229 p.

Frame, A.: A report on a pilot survey of a hospital discharge procedure, Health Bull. **26**:220-227, Oct., 1960.

Goldman, F.: Prolonged stay in general hospitals, Geriatrics **14**:789-800, Dec., 1959.

Goldmann, F., project director: The community plans for its chronically ill and aged, New York, 1961, Health Planning Committee, Council of Jewish Federations and Welfare Funds, 63 p.

Gonnerman, A. M.: After hospitalization what? Discharge planning offers answers, Hospitals **43**:81-86, April 16, 1969.

Gonnerman, A. M.: Introduction of planned discharge coordinators in hospitals, Hosp. Forum **10**:4-6, Jan., 1968.

Guiss, R.: A project to relieve overcrowding, Hosp. Community Psychiatry **19**:18-20, Jan., 1968.

Hartlage, L. C., Freeman, W., and Harine, L.: An analysis of discharge procedures, Hosp. Community Psychiatry **19**:307-310, Oct., 1968.

Hellman, L. M.: Early hospital discharge, Lancet **1**:227-232, Feb. 3, 1962.

Hicks, A. M.: Hospital helps extended care facility fulfill Medicare requirements, Hospitals **42**:53-56, Jan. 1, 1968.

Hockery, L.: Care in balance: a study of collaboration between hospital and community services, London, 1968, Queen's Institute of District Nursing, 163 p.

Horvits, D. J.: Computer simulation of hospital discharges, pub. no. 1000, series 2, no. 3, Washington, D.C., 1966, National Center for Health Statistics, Public Health Service, 35 p.

Howell, T. H.: Admissions and discharges in a geriatric unit, Hospitals **59**: 486-488, Aug., 1963.

Hunt, L. W., Zinovieff, A., and Newell, D. J.: Pre-discharge ward: a step nearer home, Nurs. Times **63**:723-725, June 2, 1967.

Jensen, F.: Medical care of the discharged hospital patient, New York, 1944, Commonwealth Fund, 94 p.

Jones, F.: Length of stay in hospital, Lancet **1**:321-323, Feb. 8, 1964.

Krueger, D., and Roberts, D.: Characteristics of long-term patients, Hospitals **30**:47-52, Aug. 1, 1956.

Kunce, J., and Anderson, W.: Maze performance and privileges in a psychiatric hospital, J. Clin. Psychol. **16**:362-364, 1960.

Lee, S.: Three-year appraisal of a hospital-home affiliation, Hospitals **42**:103-106, Aug. 16, 1968.

Leipold, W. D., and Knutson, C. S.: Differences in social desirability, anxiety, and introversion-extraversion, with varying lengths of hospitalization, Psychol. Rep. **15**:723-726, 1964.

Letourneau, C. U.: Admissions and discharges: Achilles' heel of public relations, Hosp. Manage. **92**:36-38, Sept., 1961.

Lichtenstein, M.: Length of stay and criteria for discharge in a large tuberculosis center, Am. Rev. Respir. Dis. **74**:961-963, Dec., 1956.

McGriff, D.: A coordinated approach to discharge planning, Soc. Work **10**:45-50, Jan., 1965.

Mehling, G. A.: Discharge planning for chronically ill veterans, Soc. Work **9**:79-85, July, 1964.

National Center for Health Statistics: Utilization of short-stay hospitals: summary of nonmedical statistics, United States, 1965, pub. no. 1000, series 23, no. 2, Washington, D.C., 1967, Public Health Service, 25 p.

Newell, D. J.: The predischarge ward, Lancet **2**:1293-1297, 1966.

Payson, H. E., and Davis, J. M.: The psychosocial adjustment of medical inpatients after discharge: a follow-up study, Am. J. Psychiatry **123**:1220-1225, 1967.

Pratt, R. J.: Combined admittance-discharge procedure, Hosp. Prog. **42**:58-59, June, 1961.

Pullinger, W.: A twelve-week discharge program, Hosp. Community Psychiatry **19**:21-23, Jan., 1968.

Riedel, D. C., and Fitzpatrick, T. B.: Patterns of patient care: a study of hospital use in 16 diagnoses, Ann Arbor, 1964, University of Michigan, Bureau of Hospital Administration, 292 p.

Robinson, G. H.: Prediction of hospital length of stay, Health Serv. Res. **1**:287-300, Winter, 1966.

Rosenfeld, L. S., Goldman, F., and Kaprio, L.: Reasons for prolonged hospital stay: a study of need for hospital care, J. Chronic Dis. **6**:141-152, Aug., 1957.

Rusk, H. A.: Hospital patient survey, New York, 1956, The New York Foundation, 146 p.

Slate, H.: Handling the hospital patient's ultimatum, Social Casework **39**:222-228, 1958.

Snyder, L.: The merits of discharge planning in shortening the hospitalization of free patients, Md. State Med. J. **11**:10-17, Jan., 1962.

Tedesco, J.: A study of irregular discharges in a Veterans Administration tuberculosis hospital, Am. Rev. Respir. Dis. **68**:393-399, 1953.

VanDyke, F., Brown, V., and Thom, A.: "Long" stay hospital care: reasons for prolonged stay of 611 service ward patients of all ages, hospitalized thirty days or longer in nine hospitals, municipal and voluntary, in New York City, on a census day in 1961, New York, 1963, Columbia University School of Public Health and Administrative Medicine, 112 p.

Vargas, M. J.: Departure center eases discharge, Mental Hosp. **16**:202-203, July, 1965.

Walters, R. F., and Bunch, O. E.: Utilization of provisional discharge diagnoses to enhance patient traffic-pattern studies, Med. Care **7**:313-326, July-Aug., 1969.

Wilson, M.: Follow-up study on patients discharged from a chronic disease hospital to domiciliary care during 1965 and 1966, J. Am. Geriatr. Soc. **16**:445-450, April, 1968.

Winter, K. E.: Discharge and duration of stay experience in nursing homes, J. Chronic Dis. **17**:863-878, Sept., 1964.

Witkin, M. J.: Patients discharged from short-stay hospitals, series 13, no. 4, Washington, D.C., 1965, National Center for Health Statistics, Public Health Service.

APPENDIX B

Legislation and regulations affecting discharge planning

JANET PAPILE O'DAY

Historically, health care has enjoyed relative immunity from government control and only recently has become subject to public regulation. Prior to 1965, regulation existed primarily through state licensing boards, which operated to ensure that certain health care activities met specified standards. With the passage of Medicare and Medicaid legislation, the federal government began a tenuous regulation of health care delivery to ensure that money was being spent to deliver defined services of acceptable quality to the designated population.

Since 1965, regulatory health care legislation has been created to cope with problems of recognized public concern. Administrative agencies have been expanded or established and given the responsibility for rule making in regard to specific legislation. The end result is a set of rules and regulations by which providers of health care are directed or controlled.

When one examines the effects of legislation and regulation on the discharge planning process, it becomes evident that the development of a conceptual framework is essential to place the outcomes of regulation into perspective. Table 1 illustrates the major regulatory programs that impact on the discharge planning process and highlights the principal elements of the conceptual framework that will be developed.

Legislation and the subsequent regulations in the health care industry can generally be related to three major areas of concern: access to care, quality of care, and cost of care. For example, the primary objective of Medicare was to increase access to health care for the elderly and the disabled. However, the issues of quality and cost were also addressed. Facilities and agencies were required to meet the Conditions of Participation before receiving reimbursement for services rendered. These conditions were, in effect, standards and criteria that covered many aspects of the facility's or agency's operations. Most of the Conditions of Participation pointed to quality, but some also dealt with cost. Specifically, the establishment of

Table 1. Major regulatory programs impacting on discharge planning in 1980

Origin of regulation	Source of authority	Primary intent	Impact on discharge planning process
Medicare	Federal	Access to care	Evaluate eligibility for Medicare services; determine scope of services available; assist in determination of extended stay
Medicaid	Federal/state	Access to care	Evaluate eligibility for Medicaid services; determine scope of services available; document problems with discharge planning
JCAH	Quasi-public	Quality of care	Include discharge plan in medical, nursing care, and social service plans; provide resource for health care team
PSRO	Federal/private	Cost of care	Document early discharge planning; provide certification of level of care; share information on individual cases
P.L. 93-641	Federal/state	Cost of care	Collect data on services provided, clients served, unmet needs; transform data into institutional plans
Title XX	Federal/state	Cost of care	Evaluate eligibility for Title XX services; determine scope of services in local area; articulate unmet needs

a utilization review committee (URC) was required by Medicare to review appropriateness of services and length of stay. This requirement was intended not only to ensure quality, but also to curb costs.

Few public officials anticipated the inflationary impact of Medicare legislation on the health care industry, nor did they appreciate to what extent rising costs under this program would strain the federal budget. The escalation of costs encouraged an active reexamination of the entire health care system and its regulation. One of the 1972 amendments to the Social Security Act, the Professional Standards Review Organization Amendment, extended the concept of utilization review. Judgments about appropriateness are made shortly after the time of admission and before services are provided, rather than retrospectively after a patient has been discharged and nothing can be done about inappropriateness.

Although health care costs had risen, resources had frequently been poorly allocated and in many instances inappropriately and inefficiently utilized. In 1974 the National Health Planning and Resources Development Act was enacted to improve the quality and efficiency of the health care system through planning and more rigorous controls.

Another way to view regulation is by the source of authority: federal, state, or quasi-public. Many federal health care regulations dictate what state regulations should require. States may have additional regulations not related to federal law.

The most prominent agency for quasi-public regulation of health care is the Joint Commission on the Accrediation of Hospitals (JCAH). Prior to 1965, accreditation was totally voluntary. The Medicare Conditions of Participation deemed that hospitals accredited by JCAH were eligible for Medicare reimbursement. Thus a totally voluntary program became quasi-public.

Some of the actual tasks of discharge planning have been mandated by federal, state, and quasi-public regulations. The establishment of discharge planning programs came as a direct result of some regulations and an indirect consequence of others. In some states the existence of a specific discharge planning program is mandated by state health departments (Massachusetts and New York).

In the following pages an attempt will be made to highlight the more salient health care legislation and regulations that pertain to discharge planning. Each law will be viewed in light of the source of authority, the primary intent, and the impact on the discharge planning process.

A few words must be said, at this point, regarding the roles of the discharge planning consultant and the primary provider. In many cases the primary nurse may be performing many of the tasks that have been attributed to the discharge planning consultant. In those instances the primary nurse is the discharge planner with the patient. The discharge planning consultant may function solely as a resource for the primary nurse. However, in other circumstances the discharge planning consultant may be less a resource for the primary providers and more an actual planner with the patient. How the discharge planning consultant functions and how much of the discharge planning the primary providers actually perform will vary from institution to institution and from patient to patient. The main thrust of this chapter is to illustrate the influence of regulations on the process of discharge planning.

MEDICARE

Origin of regulation

Title XVIII, a 1965 amendment to the Social Security Act, established what is commonly known as Medicare. This is a two-part health insurance program for the elderly and disabled. Part A provides hospital insurance benefits and is financed through hospital insurance taxes. Part B, Supplementary Medical Insurance Benefits, covers the cost of physician services and a number of other items and services not covered under Part A. Part B is optional and is financed through monthly premiums from enrollees and matching contributions from the federal government. The 1972 amendments to the Social Security Act allow for automatic enrollment in Part B for all persons eligible for Part A unless the person specifies otherwise.

Source of authority

Medicare is administered through the federal government. The passage of Title XVIII required that Congress assign to the Social Security Administration the task of rule making and standard setting for the health care industry. The Social Security Administration assumed the responsibility for developing the mechanical procedures and policies used to monitor provider compliance. In 1977 the Social Security Administration was incorporated into a new organizational structure within the Department of Health, Education, and Welfare: the Health Care Financing Administration.

Primary intent

The goal of the Medicare program was to decrease the financial barriers to health care for the elderly and disabled. Specifically, benefits for hospital, nursing home, and home health care were offered to the elderly and disabled. The attendant regulations included specific requirements that determined eligibility for those benefits as well as the scope of services allowed.

Impact

Under Medicare the major task for discharge planners is to understand the regulations and to be able to apply the most recent criteria espoused in the Medicare handbooks to patients in need of discharge planning. Skilled and restorative services must be provided either in Medicare-participating extended care facilities or by certified home health agencies. One of the major problems in discharge planning is that many elderly and disabled patients do require postdischarge care, but such care is neither restorative nor skilled as defined by Medicare. Much of the discharge planner's time and energy is therefore directed toward educating other providers, as well as patients and families, as to which postdischarge services are covered. Published information can be misleading. For example, statements such as, "Medicare will pay for up to 100 days of extended care only after the patient has been hospitalized for three days," have led to false assumptions by some patients. Hospitalization for three days does not guarantee Medicare reimbursement for long-term care unless the patient requires Medicare-defined skilled or restorative care. Even when care is covered, the coverage does not necessarily last for 100 days or 100 visits, but only as long as the patient continues to require skilled services.

The discharge planning consultant, together with the other health care team members, determines the need for postdischarge Medicare-covered services. The implementation of discharge plans is possible only when there is a Medicare-certified agency or facility available to provide the required services. It is the responsibility of the discharge planning consultant to be aware of all possible community services and to recommend an appropriate facility or agency to the primary provider and the patient.

The discharge planning consultant has an additional responsibility for Medicare patients requiring discharge planning. In the utilization review process of determination of extended stay, the need for continued hospitalization is based first on the need for continued hospital level of care (which includes daily medical treatment) and second on the need for placement in a Medicare-defined level of extended care. Progress with discharge plans must be communicated to the health care team and the utilization review committee (URC) to ensure that the hospital will be paid for that period while the patient is awaiting placement in a Medicare-covered facility.

MEDICAID

Origin of regulation

Title XIX, an additional 1965 amendment to the Social Security Act, provides grants to the states for their medical assistance programs. The purpose of this amendment, popularly called Medicaid, is to enable states to furnish medical benefits to the aged, blind, and disabled, and to families with dependent children whose income and resources are insufficient to pay for necessary medical and rehabilitative services.

Source of authority

Medicaid is a joint federal and state program. If a state chooses to participate in the program, coverage of certain "categorically needy" persons is required, whereas coverage of other "categorically needy" and "medically needy" persons is optional. Each state is given considerable latitude by the federal government to determine the scope of services to be provided and the eligibility requirements.

Primary intent

The primary intent of Medicaid is to give the needy access to health care. Medicaid provides benefits for those defined as eligible by the federal and state governments. Because the federal and state governments are buying certain services, the agencies and facilities certified to provide these services must meet minimum standards as defined by the Medicaid regulations. Such Medicaid Conditions of Participation deal primarily with quality of care.

Impact

To make determinations about an appropriate plan of aftercare, the discharge planner must have a working knowledge of the local Medicaid program. The discharge planner should be informed about both the financial and the social eligibility requirements for medical assistance. If a patient is eligible to receive benefits but is not yet enrolled as a recipient of a medical assistance program, it is sometimes essential that enrollment be accomplished before the most appropriate discharge plan can be implemented. This is especially true for the patient who cannot return home for health and social reasons. The home situation may be unsafe, or the patient may require 24-hour care and supervision. Therefore placement in an intermediate care facility covered only by Medicaid may be necessary.

Many of the bureaucratic problems that discharge planners and patients face in regard to Medicaid vary from state to state. The specific effects of Medicaid on the discharge planning process will also depend on the state's program. The major point to be remembered is that discharge planners have a responsibility to be aware of the local Medicaid program so that it can be used effectively for discharge planning.

JOINT COMMISSION ON THE ACCREDITATION OF HOSPITALS

Origin of regulation

The Joint Commission on the Accreditation of Hospitals (JCAH) is a private, nonprofit organization. Review by the JCAH establishes that a facility has voluntarily chosen to be measured against standards developed by the commission. These standards apply to the overall operation of a facility and measure the performance of each of its functions.

Source of authority

As previously mentioned, JCAH activities do relate to various government mandates, thus giving it a quasi-public authority.

Primary intent

The primary purpose of the JCAH is to promote quality in the provision of health care. Accreditation by the JCAH developed from the desire of surgeons, and later hospital administrators, to comply voluntarily with minimum standards by which to judge their services to both the patients and the community.

Impact

Continuity of care is an underlying theme of the JCAH professional practice standards. The JCAH requires that the medical and nursing plans of care be coordinated with each other and include discharge plans. The standards encourage liaison with community agencies or facilities to ensure continuity of care from the hospital to the patient's home or another facility. Actual measurement of the implementation of these standards requires that there be written evidence of discharge plans in the medical record and the nursing Kardex. In addition, the institution may be asked to produce a documented program for discharge planning.

The JCAH promotes a team approach to discharge planning. This team includes at least the physician and the nurse but also may include the social worker, dietitian, therapists, and other professionals involved in the care of the patient. The discharge planning program enhances this approach through additional coordination and communication between the facility and the community.

PROFESSIONAL STANDARDS REVIEW ORGANIZATIONS

Origin of regulation

The 1972 amendments to the Social Security Act included the professional standards review organization program, commonly known as PSRO. The legislation provides for the establishment of PSROs that are charged with reviewing appropriateness and quality of medical services provided within their designated geographic areas to beneficiaries of the Social Security Act. The PSROs have been encouraged to delegate responsibility for reviews to institutions that have demonstrated the ability to conduct adequate reviews. The reviews include admission certification of institutional services, periodic sample reviews by diagnosis or condition, regular reviews of patient and provider profiles, and monitoring of the certification requirements of the Social Security Administration.

Source of authority

The Department of Health, Education, and Welfare (DHEW) has contracted with private medical care foundations, which are local corporations run by physicians, to conduct the designated reviews. In essence, DHEW is attempting to monitor and evaluate performance by contract. The PSRO legislation does authorize the establishment of state PSRO councils in any state with three or more PSROs. The state councils coordinate and integrate the activities of the various PSROs, serve as an appeal agent, and assist the secretary of DHEW in the conduct of the program. The determinations of PSROs are conclusive for payment purposes.

Primary intent

The explicit objectives of the PSRO legislation address the necessity for institutional admission, the duration of institutional care, and the adequacy and relevance of the service provided. The implied objectives include cost control of federal health care services and the assurance that services rendered are medically necessary and appropriate. The primary intent of the law is to limit the growth of Medicare and Medicaid spending without forcing medical standards below an acceptable level.

Impact

The PSROs have affected discharge planning in several ways. Some discharge planning consultants actually function not only as discharge planners but also as PSRO coordinators, performing admission reviews and extended stay reviews. Where the discharge planning consultant is not the PSRO coordinator, it is essential that a close working relationship develop between the PRSO and the discharge planning program. This is particularly crucial in extended stay reviews when a hospital patient is awaiting placement in a Medicare-covered facility. The primary provider or the discharge planning consultant must have documented, in the medical record and on a regularly scheduled basis, a discharge planning note that outlines the plan and goals for the patient and the recommended level of care. This documentation allows the PSRO coordinators to determine that discharge planning has been instituted, available resources have been identified for postdischarge care, and progress toward obtaining postdischarge care has been made.

In most institutions, the PSRO and the URC have merged. The PSRO has adopted standards and criteria based on typical patterns of medical practice in the region, so that the appropriateness of utilization and the quality of institutional services can be evaluated. This leaves, for the URC, discussion of only those cases that fall outside the norm. It is essential that not only the PSRO coordinator but also the discharge planning consultant (if a different individual) participate in the URC. The information that the discharge planner has gathered during the assessment phase of the discharge planning process cannot alter the level of aftercare needed, but sharing this information with URC does afford the opportunity to elicit medical and administrative support for the necessary discharge plan.

For example, a patient whose extended stay falls outside the ninetieth percentile may be discussed at a URC meeting in accordance with the hospital's utilization review plan. The discharge planner has determined that this patient does not require placement in a Medicare-covered facility. The URC may further clarify the medical plan regarding the patient's hospital course and either concur with the discharge planner's determination or assist in the establishment of a new plan of aftercare. This activity is essential in judging when to terminate or reinstate Medicare benefits.

Thus one of the responsibilities of the PSRO is the determination of the required level of care for patients. Assessment of level of care for discharge planning has been the discharge planning consultant's responsibility since the inception of Medicare and Medicaid. Once a patient no longer requires an acute hospital level of care (as determined by the PSRO physician and the attending physician), it is essential to determine whether the patient requires the Medicare-covered level of extended care. Otherwise, Medicare benefits must be terminated by the PSRO, or the institution will risk the loss of Medicare certification.

PUBLIC LAW 93-641

Origin of regulation

The National Health Planning and Resources Development Act of 1974, commonly known as Public Law 93-641, provides a system of procedures to effect the goals of both the development and allocation of health services based on statistical profile of present and potential community health patterns and care needs. An additional principle built into the law is that planning should be done primarily by consumers, together with representatives of providers and private agencies.

Source of authority

The actual authority to implement the congressional purposes of this law is vested in state and regional entities. Public Law 93-641 established new state agencies, the state health planning and development agencies (SHPDAs), and quasi public regional agencies, the health systems agencies (HSAs) and the statewide health coordinating councils (SHCCs). The HSAs are designated by the secretary of DHEW to perform health planning and regulatory functions. The statement of desired improvements in the health status of the area population and in the agencies serving the population should be expressed in a health systems plan (HSP) and an annual implementation plan (AIP).

The governor of each state selects the members of the SHPDA. This agency is responsible for the preparation of an administrative program to execute the legislative responsibilities of the state. In addition, the SHCC, composed of members also appointed by the governor of the state, must have 60% representation from the HSAs and 50% consumer representation. The SHCC is responsible for the adoption of the state health plan (SHP), the review of HSA budgets, and the provision of council to the SHPDA on the performance of its functions. The SHP is a compilation of the health systems plans, which are modified if necessary by the SHPDA and approved by the SHCC.

Primary intent

The primary intent of Public Law 93-641 is to do more with less and to use what is available effectively. The HSA is expected to develop a health systems plan that delineates priorities among stated goals and objectives and recommends changes in the health care system. The implementation of the plan will be partially accomplished by reviewing facility and service plans against the state health plan. To support applications and obtain required approval, health care providers must justify, with comprehensive documentation, the demand for any planned or desired new service, as well as demonstrate its financial feasibility. Providers have become active in the planning process not only to meet the requirements of the law but also to have meaningful input into the planning agencies.

Impact

Discharge planning is greatly affected by a state's health systems plan. In states with mandated institutional long-range plans, it is essential that each institution's needs in terms of discharge planning be articulated in its one- and five-year plans, so that each area health plan will in turn reflect these needs.

Each discharge planner keeps statistics of varying kinds related to the number of referrals and types of services, but there is no uniform system of reporting that would make these numbers significant. Discharge planning programs respond on a demand basis to queries by state health agencies regarding numbers of patients awaiting placement in a facility or remaining at home with services provided.

Planning as a management technique in discharge planning is critical and now has a vehicle for implementation. Discharge planning programs ought to be submitting one- and five-year plans to their institutions. These plans should be based on the discharge planning consultant's experience as well as on the medical needs of the service area's projected population. For example, if the majority of patients who have needed discharge planning and subsequent long-term care are elderly but the number of elderly admissions to the institution and concurrently the number of elderly in the institution's service area are decreasing, this situation must be addressed in the long-term plans of the discharge planning program and the institution. The focus of the health plans may need to change from an emphasis on increasing long-term care services for the elderly to perhaps better integration of already existing services.

Data from the discharge planning consultants of hospitals and long-term care facilities have key information that ought to be included in a health systems plan and a state health plan. Each discharge planning consultant has the responsibility to try to help the HSAs effect change that is in keeping with the genuine needs of the consumers they serve.

TITLE XX

Origin of regulation

Title XX refers to the 1975 Social Services Amendment to the Social Security Act. The overall goal of Title XX is to allow the states to define the content and nature of their social services delivery system within broadly defined requirements. Citizen participation and review are mandated. In theory the content of each state's Title XX plan is subject to the approval of the state's citizens rather than the approval of the federal government. To achieve the Title XX goals, local government, interested organizations, and concerned citizens can help determine which services to offer, which people to serve, and how to divide the funds among geographic areas, services, and groups that need help.

Source of authority

The federal government established guidelines that the states must follow within their service plans. Any social services provided under Title XX must be directed to at least one of the federally specified goals, and one service must be directed to all the goals. These goals are generally geared toward self-sufficiency, protection, and appropriate use of institutions. In addition, the federal government has indicated broad eligibility requirements. Every year each state must formulate a comprehensive social services plan that includes the federal goals and eligibility requirements.

Primary intent

The primary intent of Title XX is cost related, with increased social service provision for the "categorically needy." Each state is awarded a finite number of dollars with which to implement the social services plan. Citizen participation is intended to ensure that the finite resources will be distributed throughout the states according to the perceived needs of the population and through an acceptable political process.

Impact

The discharge planner should be aware of the local Title XX plan, and the Title XX services should be included in the array of resources available to patients after discharge. Social services and health services frequently overlap. For example, homemaking is a social service as defined by the federal government and may be included in the Title XX service plan. A homemaker's duties include cleaning, washing, food shopping, and meal preparation. A patient who is newly discharged from an institution may require this service during the recuperative period. The social service required has been dictated not only by the patient's social situation but also by the patient's health condition. This patient may also have a need for continued nursing or medical services. It is the the discharge planning consultant who must facilitate the coordination of the social and health services needed to ensure appropriate postdischarge care.

Discharge planning consultants have an additional responsibility under Title XX. Either as a concerned citizen or as a member of an organization of professionals, the discharge planner has a duty to convey to the Title XX planners the social service needs of the patients who require discharge planning from hospitals and other institutions. The federal mandate dictates this kind of input, and the states need assistance to determine which services to provide for whom. The discharge planning consultant can give invaluable assistance to the states by providing statistical data and other information that presents the needs of persons being discharged from hospitals and institutions or of persons who are never discharged due to lack of appropriate services in the community.

REGULATIONS IN ACTION: A CASE EXAMPLE

For a clarification of the conceptual framework, it may be helpful to look at an actual case study and analyze the regulatory influences on the outcome of the discharge planning. The case is not a model of how discharge planning should proceed but rather an illustration of the influences of regulations on the final outcome. Table 2 analyzes the chronological events in the case in relation to the regulations, their primary intent, and their impact on the discharge planning process.

Case study. Ms. B., a 93-year-old single woman, was admitted to the hospital on June 11 with a chief complaint of anorexia. On June 19 Ms. B. was referred to the discharge planning unit by the physician. At this time it was determined by the physician that the patient was receiving the acute hospital level of care. The physician continued to perform diagnostic tests to confirm a suspected carcinoma. A family conference was scheduled by the discharge planner for June 20 because both the physician and the discharge planner believed that this patient would require extensive discharge planning.

Ms. B. had been living with an elderly niece and nephew for the previous five years. Prior to that time she had lived and worked in a rectory. She had never before been hospitalized. The nephew had become seriously ill about six months previously. At that time Ms. B. signed over most of her money to the niece and nephew to defray some of the medical expenses. The niece and nephew reported that Ms. B.'s behavior changed shortly after her money was transferred. She became confused and forgetful.

At the time of the family conference, Ms. B. was receiving intravenous therapy and was recovering from aspiration pneumonia and an allergic reaction to antibiotics. In addition, she had lower intestine bleeding and anemia. She was disoriented, confused, and was pulling out her intravenous equipment. She required frequent nursing care to be fed, washed, turned, and kept dry. Her prognosis was poor, but it was difficult to determine the outcome at this point.

It was necessary to discuss finances with the niece and nephew to determine what resources were already available to Ms. B. and what might still be needed. Because Ms. B.'s only monthly income was

Table 2. Impact of regulations in case example

Event	Regulation	Primary intent	Impact on discharge planning
Referral to discharge planner	JCAH PSRO	Quality Cost	*As intended* Discharge planning part of patient care plan and identified early
Assessment of required level of care	PSRO Medicare	Cost Access	*As intended* Evaluation of level of care to determine necessity for Medicare to pay for hospitalization
Determination of available resources	Medicare Medicaid Title XX	Access Access Cost	*As intended* Discharge planner able to evaluate eligibility for all possible discharge plans
Application for Medicaid	Medicaid	Access	*As intended* But with long delay awaiting approval
Assessment of required level of aftercare	PSRO Medicare Medicaid	Cost Access Access	*As intended* Discharge planner required to document level of care and action on discharge plan on a regularly scheduled basis
Termination of Medicare benefits; reinstatement; retermination	Medicare PSRO	Access Cost	*As intended* Discharge planner interprets ramifications of termination and reinstatement process, and works with fiscal department and Medicaid to ensure payment for discharge plan
Delay in placement	P.L. 93-641	Cost	*Opposite effect* Shortage of available nursing home beds (SHP does not call for more beds but rather community alternatives)
Placement in nursing home	Medicaid	Access	*As intended*

her Social Security check, and it appeared that her other assets amounted to very little, it was decided that application for medical assistance would be made. The application was completed on June 25.

Under Medicare, Ms. B. might be eligible for visiting nurse and home health aide services for a short period of time. Under Title XX, Ms. B. might be eligible for up to 20 hours of homemaker time per week. However, due to the disability of the nephew, the ages of the niece and nephew, and the current status of Ms. B., home care of any kind did not seem appropriate. Other alternatives to nursing home placement, such as day care or foster home care, were not available in Ms. B.'s community. If Ms. B. were to be placed in a nursing home, she might be eligible for Medicare coverage. However, if she were to remain in the nursing home once she no longer needed a skilled level of care, there would be no resources to pay the nursing home. If at the time of discharge from the hospital she did not meet Medicare eligibility requirements for skilled care, there would be no resources to pay the nursing home initially. Medicaid in Ms. B.'s state would pay for nursing home care as well as visiting nurse and home health aide services once Medicare no longer paid.

The initial application for Medicaid was denied on July 25 because the cash-in value of a life insurance policy plus the amount of money still in the savings account was equal to slightly more than the amount of assets allowed by the state for Medicaid eligibility. The processing of Medicaid applications in Ms. B.'s state generally takes four to six weeks. During the time a Medicaid application is pending, it is not possible to find an available nursing home bed because the private nursing homes need to be assured that they will receive payment for services rendered. Medicaid approval pending is no guarantee of payment, and private nursing homes will not take referrals on these patients. In Ms. B.'s state there are no state or municipal nursing homes—only private ones.

By July 28, Ms. B.'s condition improved to the point where she was continent, ambulatory with the assistance of one person, independemt in washing and dressing, and only slightly confused. Hospital Medicare benefits were terminated by PSRO/URC. On August 14, Ms. B. developed a urinary tract infection with an elevated temperature, and hospital Medicare benefits were reinstated. On August 31 the infection had been resolved, and hospital Medicare benefits were again terminated.

The surplus assets that were the cause of Ms. B.'s ineligibility for Medicaid were utilized to pay for the days of hospitalization that accumulated after Medicare benefits had been terminated. Once that money was paid to the hospital, a copy of the receipt was sent to the Medicaid division of the welfare department, and the Medicaid application was reactivated. A Medicaid approval was issued on August 30.

The primary providers spoke to the niece and nephew frequently during this time. The nephew was failing rapidly, and the niece was caring for him at home. Even though Ms. B. had improved significantly, the family could not care for her at home. This problem was thoroughly discussed with Ms. B., who agreed that placement in a nursing home was the best solution. Because Ms. B. had improved, she no longer required the Medicare-defined level of skilled care. She was discharged to an intermediate care facility, covered by Medicaid in her state, on November 8.

The discharge planning consultant had actively looked for an available bed in an appropriate facility for over two months. The HSA of that particular area had determined that there are more nursing home beds in the area than are needed, based on the present and projected population. According to the HSA planning formula, this is in fact true. However, the dilemma remains that it is difficult to find available beds. The area has yet to develop community alternatives so that more nursing home beds are made available. Until this is accomplished, finding available nursing home beds for such patients as Ms. B. will continue to be difficult and time consuming.

CONCLUSION

It is clear that many regulations (based on legislation related to Medicare, Medicaid, JCAH, PSRO, Public Law 93-461, and Title XX) must be understood before discharge planning can be effective. The discharge planner has the responsibility to satisfy the regulations by combining relevant legal requirements with individual patient needs to maximize appropriate access and quality at the least cost. The case example illustrates the complexity of this responsibility. Regulations frequently overlap and make discharge planning tasks duplicative and time consuming.

When the regulations are understood in terms of the primary intent of the legislation, it is easier to see that regulations are not barriers to providing quality care. The discharge planner must regard regulations as tools for implementing the primary intent of the legislation and learn to make them work for the discharge planning process.

ACKNOWLEDGMENT

I would like to thank Mark D. Mandel, former Director of Regulatory Activities, Boston University Center for Health Planning, for his guidance in the development of this paper.

ADDITIONAL READINGS

Affeldt, J. E.; JCAH: the best game in town, Hosp. Prog. **59**: 51-54, Sept., 1978.

Blum, J. D., Gertman, P. M., and Rabinow, J.; PSROs and the law, Germantown, M., 1977, Aspen Systems Corp.

Commerce Clearing House; 1974 Social Security and Medicare explained, Chicago, 1974. Commerce Clearing House.

Dallas, J. L.; The HSA and the PSRO: toward a linkage, Public Health Rep. **91**:46-50, Jan.-Feb., 1976.

Decker, B., and Bonner, P., editors: *PSRO:* organization for regional peer review, Cambridge, Mass., 1973, Ballinger Publishing Co.

Health Planning Council of Greater Boston: Health Planning and Resource Development Act of 1974, Boston, 1974, the Council.

Havighurst, C., and Blumstein, J. F.: Coping with quality/cost trade-offs in medical care: the role of the PSROs, Northwestern Univ. Law Rev., vol. 70, no. 1, 1975.

Leone, R. A.: The real costs of regulation, Harvard Bus. Rev., pp. 57-66, Nov.-Dec., 1977.

Mandel, M. D.: New opportunities for the public to shape the nation's institutional health services, Am. J. Law Med. **3**:49-57, 1977.

Noll, R. G.: Reforming regulation: an evaluation of the Ash Council proposals, Washington, D.C., 1971, The Brookings Institution.

Mantis, C. A.: PSRO coordination—is it nursing? Am. J. Nurs. **78**:1534-1535, Sept., 1978.

Palmer, R. E.: The march of history: growing regulations and growing costs, Hosp. Prog. **59**:58-61, Sept., 1978.

Somers, A. R.: Hospital regulation: the dilemma of public policy, Princeton, N.J. 1969, Princeton University.

Somers, H. M., and Somers, A. R.: Medicare and the hospitals: issues and prospects, Washington, D.C., 1967, The Brookings Institution.

Stephenson, G. W.: At hand: bureaucratic surveillance, Hosp. Prog. **59**:50-51, Sept., 1978.

APPENDIX C

Regulations governing continuing care services in [Massachusetts] hospitals

The Department of Public Health, acting under authority of Massachusetts General Laws, Chapter 111, Section 53, and every other act thereto enabling, hereby establishes an amendment to "Licensure Rules and Regulations for Hospitals in Massachusetts" to govern Continuing Care Services in Hospitals. Said additional section was approved and adopted by the Department of Public Health on August 10, 1971, and filed on August 13, 1971, with the Secretary of State to be effective the date of publication by the Secretary.

1.0 Planning for continuing care

There shall be an organized multidisciplinary service to aid the attending physician and his patient in planning for continuing care upon discharge from the hospital. The continuing care service shall be designed so as to facilitate the transfer of the patient from the hospital setting to an appropriate independent living arrangement or to another institution or level of care therein.

1.1 The hospital administrator in conjunction with the Directors of Nursing and Social Service shall designate a specific individual to be known as the "Coordinator of Continuing Care" or designate a specific unit for this purpose.

1.1.1 Wherever an individual is designated as the "Coordinator of Continuing Care," the individual shall be a *social worker or public health nurse* [italics added] and shall have particular competence in carrying out this responsibility based on education, experience, and knowledge of community resources.

1.1.2 Wherever a specific unit is designated, there shall be at least a nurse and social worker assigned to the unit to assess patient needs and to plan together for continuity of patient care.

1.2 The coordinator shall be responsible for the coordination of the plan for continuing care under the direction of the physician and in cooperation with the patient, the family, and other members of the professional staff.

1.3 A mechanism shall be established, operative and described in writing, for early screening of patients to determine whether continuing care planning will be necessary.

1.4 The individual or unit responsible for coordination of planning for continuing care shall maintain in writing a current description of out-of-hospital resources which shall be available to the attending physician and other members of the professional staff.

1.5 The Coordinator of Continuing Care shall be responsible for the timely transfer of appropriate information from the hospital to the posthospital institution or agency in order to insure continuity of patient care.

1.5.1 When a patient is transferred to another institution, a patient care referral form approved by the Department shall be completed and accompany the patient.

1.5.2 When a patient is discharged and referred to a community agency for continuing care, a patient care referral form approved by the Department shall be completed and sent to the agency prior to, or at the time of, patient discharge.

1.5.3 The medical discharge summary shall be sent by the hospital no later than 72 hours following discharge of the patient to an institution or community agency.

1.6 The hospital shall give notice of anticipated or impending transfer of the patient to the community agency or institution at least 24 hours prior to discharge and shall assist in making arrangements for safe transportation.

1.7 The coordinator shall assist the utilization review committee in its consideration of the appropriateness of continuity of patient care.

1.8 Written records shall be maintained which contain sufficient information to enable the coordinator or unit to prepare periodic reports which shall include the number of patients for whom coordination of continuing care was provided and the types of placement made.

Index

CONTINUING CARE

A multidisciplinary approach to discharge planning